REVISITING ANTENATAL CARE

Discover Why First Trimester is the True Foundation of a Healthy Pregnancy and How Early Action Can Change Everything

DR. DINESH KANFADE

Copyright @ 2025 by Dr. Dinesh Kanfade

All rights reserved. No part of this book may be reproduced in any form without the permission in writing from the author.

No part of this publication may be reproduced or transmitted in any form or by any means, mechanical or electronic, including photocopying or recording or by any information storage and retrieval system or transmitted by email or by any other means whatsoever without permission in writing from the author.

Disclaimer:

While the publisher and author have used their best efforts in preparing this book, they make no representation or warranties with respect to the accuracy or completeness of the contents of this book and specifically disclaim any implied warranties of merchantability or fitness for a particular purpose. No warranty may be created or extended by sales representatives or written sales materials. The advice and strategies contained herein may not be suitable for your situation. This book is for educational purpose only. It is not intended for the substitute for the diagnosis, treatment and advice of a qualified licensed professional. You should consult your healthcare provider for individualized advice. Neither the publisher nor the author shall be liable for any other commercial damages, including but not limited to special, incidental, consequential, personal, or other damage.

ACKNOWLEDGEMENTS

I wish to express my gratitude to various sources, knowingly or unknowingly has contributed for empowering my knowledge, empowering women's health and helping me to write this book.

Book Content Sources Credit and Courtesy: *

I am also grateful to the **medical community and thought leaders** whose research, insights, and innovations have contributed to the evolving understanding of antenatal care—especially in its most critical **preconceptional and first trimester phase.**

I would like to thank my mentors and teachers who had been a torch bearer for me for writing this book.

I am extremely thankful to **Dr. M. G. Sawant,** Consultant Obstetrician & Gynecologist for taking time from his busy schedule to write **"FOREWORD"** for my book.

I also express my sincere gratitude to my family members and friends who have always been supportive and motivated me in my initiatives in writing series of books on **"Women's Health"**, this book being 12th in the series.

DEDICATION

Dedicated to my better half Nita,

son Akshay, daughter-in-law Priya

and little sweet Avni.

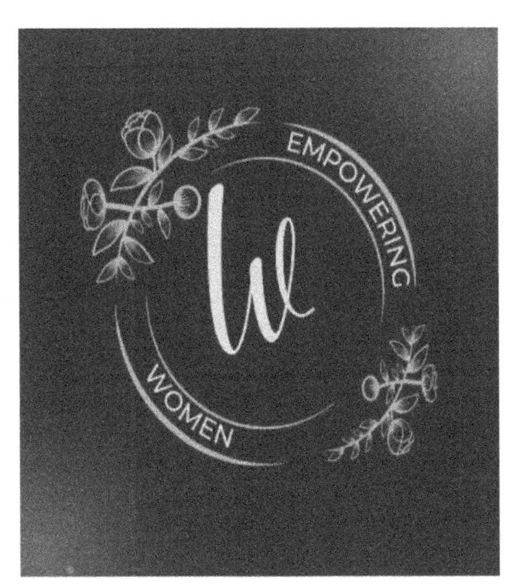

EMPOWERING
WOMEN

"We don't just need more antenatal care.

We need earlier, smarter,

and more human antenatal care."

-Anonymous

"The more we know early in pregnancy, the better we can plan and prevent complications. Knowledge is the first step towards a safer pregnancy."

-Anonymous

FOREWORD

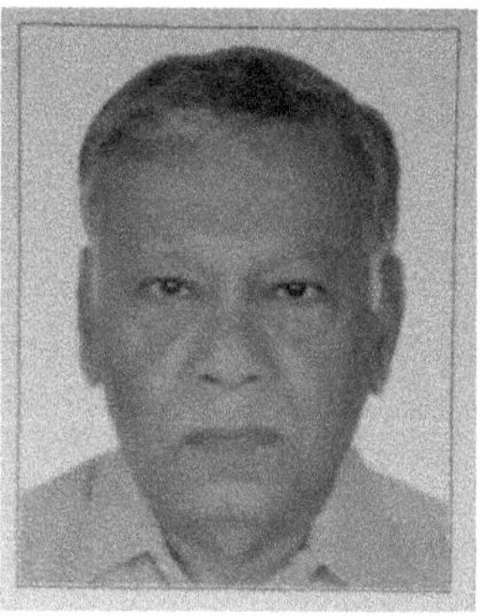

When the author first shared the vision behind this book, I immediately knew it was both **timely and necessary**. As practicing Obstetricians and Gynecologists, we witness firsthand the profound impact that early antenatal care—or the lack thereof—can have on maternal and fetal outcomes.

In many parts of the world, especially in resource-limited settings, antenatal care continues to follow an outdated pattern: the first visit happens too late, essential screenings are delayed, and the **most critical window—the first trimester**—is often overlooked. **But science tells us otherwise.** The earliest weeks of pregnancy lay the foundation for everything - from organ development and maternal adaptation to the prevention of complications.

Antenatal care is often seen as a routine checklist of scans and supplements, but what if the true foundation of a healthy pregnancy begins far earlier than we act? *Revisiting Antenatal Care* redefines conventional prenatal care by shining a spotlight on the most overlooked yet critical period—**the preconceptional and the first trimester.** First trimester is the period of **organogenesis**, and if any insult occurs in this phase, there is **likelihood of teratogenesis** in the developing fetus. Backed by scientific evidence and enriched with clinical insights, this book challenges outdated approaches and brings a new lens to pregnancy care, advocating for timely education, personalized screenings, and early emotional and physical support.

Revisiting Antenatal Care is a powerful call to rethink, redesign, and realign our approach. What makes this book stand out is its **blend of medical insight and compassionate perspective**. It offers evidence-based strategies, highlights global best practices, and addresses real-world implementation challenges—while keeping the woman at the center of care.

I commend the author for bringing clarity, structure, and heart to this often-neglected topic. The chapters are thoughtfully organized, and the language is accessible without compromising scientific accuracy—making this book equally valuable for professionals, students, and public health advocates.

It is an honor to write this foreword, and an even greater privilege to witness the impact this book is bound to make.

With admiration and support,

DR. M. G. SAWANT
MD., DGO., DFP.
Consultant Obstetrician & Gynecologist
Ex-Unit Head, Department of Obstetrics & Gynecology
E.S.I.S. Group of Hospitals Mumbai.

PREFACE

The idea for this book was born out of a simple yet persistent question I kept asking myself as a healthcare professional: **"Why do we continue to place most of our antenatal focus so late in pregnancy—when so much could have been done early on?"**

Over the years, I have witnessed the joy of healthy deliveries and the heartbreak of complications that could have been prevented—if only the right care had reached the mother at the right time. The more I studied, the more I realized that **our antenatal care model needed to be turned on its head**. What we treat as the "early phase" is, in fact, the **true foundation of pregnancy health**.

This book, ***Revisiting Antenatal Care***, is an attempt to spark that much-needed shift in perception and practice. It invites us to stop viewing the first trimester as a passive waiting period and start treating it as a **powerful window of prevention, education, and transformation**.

I have written this book for:

- Clinicians and healthcare workers who want to do more than follow routine protocols;
- Medical students seeking a deeper understanding of patient-centered antenatal care;
- Public health professionals working to build more effective maternal health systems;
- And most importantly, for the countless women who deserve to be **informed, empowered, and supported** from the very beginning of their pregnancy journey.

This is not a textbook. It is a blend of **science, strategy, and heart**—written in a way that bridges medical accuracy with real-life challenges. It draws from international guidelines, emerging innovations, and on-the-ground realities, especially in developing regions.

As you turn these pages, I hope you'll discover not just information—but inspiration. Let us revisit antenatal care—not to criticize, but to evolve. Let us shift the spotlight—**from reaction to readiness, from late action to early empowerment.**

Because when we change how we begin, we can change everything that follows.

Warm regards,

DR. DINESH KANFADE
MBBS., DGO., DFP., FICMCH., CIMP.
Sr. Obstetrician & Gynecologist
Author & Advocate for Women's Health

TABLE OF CONTENT

INTRODUCTION 15

CHAPTER I: THE EVOLUTION OF ANTENATAL CARE... 17

(A)Ancient Beginnings: Care Rooted in Tradition.......... 17

(B)Traditional Approach to ANC 20

(C)Reducing Congenital Birth Defects through Preconception and Early Pregnancy Care 23

(D)The Crucial Role of Preconception and Early Antenatal Screening – A case of Thalassemia 28

CHAPTER II: PRECONCEPTIONAL COUNSELING 35

(A) Importance of Preconceptional Care/Visit 35

(B) Identifying and Managing Chronic Conditions.......... 39

(C) Nutritional Advice and Lifestyle Modifications......... 43

(D) Genetic Counseling and Family History 49

(E)Vaccination and Infection Screening Before Conception 60

(F) Medication Review of Existing Diseases and Risk Modifications Before Pregnancy 64

(G) Challenges / Obstacles in Preconceptional Care........ 67

CHAPTER III: FIRST TRIMESTER: THE CRITICAL WINDOW 69

(A) Milestones in First Trimester Development............... 69

(B) First Trimester Screening and Investigations — and Therefore the Importance of Early Booking 73

(C) The Role of Nutrition and Supplementation — In General and in Relation to Organogenesis and Teratogenic Risk.. 76

CHAPTER IV: EARLY RISK STRATIFICATION........ 82

(A) Advanced Screening Protocols 82

(B) The Latest Predictive Markers for Preeclampsia, GDM, and Aneuploidies 104

(C) How to Design Personalized Care Pathways for Better Pregnancy Outcomes.. 118

CHAPTER V: SAFE MEDICATIONS AND SUPPLEMENTS 124

(A) First Checkpoint: Securing the Medication Landscape 124

(B) Category-Wise Drug Safety in Pregnancy 130

(C) Foundations of a Healthy Beginning: Essential Supplements for the First Trimester 133

CHAPTER VI: NAVIGATING NUTRITION PITFALLS AND RISKY HABITS IN EARLY PREGNANCY....... 137

(A) Busting Dietary Myths of the First Trimester 137

(B) Silent Threats: Alcohol, Tobacco/Smoking, and Environmental Hazards 141

(C) Cultural Beliefs and Religious Practices: Respecting Traditions While Safeguarding Health 144

CHAPTER VII: EMOTIONAL WELLNESS IN PREGNANCY: COUNSELING, SCREENING & SUPPORT 148

(A) Building Emotional Readiness for Parenthood........ 148

(B) Mental Health Checkpoints in Antenatal Care......... 151

(C) The Power of Together: Partner and Family Support in Pregnancy 154

CHAPTER VIII: COMMUNICATION: EMPOWERING WOMEN WITH KNOWLEDGE 157

(A) Patient Education Strategies: Bridging the Gap Between Clinicians and Expectant Women 157

(B) Guidelines and Recommendations: FIGO, ACOG, WHO — What They Say About Early Antenatal Care... 160

(C) Challenges in Implementation: The Roadblocks in Developing Countries 163

(D) The Future of Early Antenatal Care: Innovation, Integration, and Inclusion 166

CHAPTER IX: CONCLUSION: STRONG BEGINNINGS, SAFER JOURNEY 169

CHAPTER X: REFERENCES 171

Previous Books Published in the Series, "Women's Health" 179

INTRODUCTION

"This book invites us to stop viewing the first trimester as a passive waiting period but start treating it as a powerful window of prevention, education, and transformation."

In the ever-evolving landscape of obstetric care, the traditional model of antenatal check-ups – primarily focused on the later stages of pregnancy – no longer suffices. The modern understanding of fetal development, maternal health, and disease prevention demands a paradigm shift in our approach to antenatal care. This book *"Revisiting Antenatal Care"* introduces and explores the concepts, where the emphasis moves from late-term management towards early identification, intervention and education.

Why this Book???

Pregnancy is a physiological journey, but it can become pathological in the absence of timely care. Many complications that arise in the second and third trimesters have their origins in the earliest weeks – or even before conception. This book underlines a need to redefine ANC by recognizing the first trimester and preconceptional period as the most crucial windows for screening, prevention and risk stratification.

Modern advances in diagnostics, genetics, and maternal medicine enable us to detect high-risk conditions early, modify risk factors, switch medications that could harm the fetus, and counsel women about lifestyle and nutritional choices that directly affect fetal organogenesis. Yet, despite the evidence, a disproportionate amount of focus in clinical practice still lies in final trimester. The goal of this book is to correct this imbalance and offer a structured, evidence-based approach that aligns with contemporary research and clinical priorities.

Who is this book for???

Healthcare Providers: Obstetricians, general practitioners, nurses, midwives, and healthcare policymakers will get practical guidance in implementing early ANC protocols and improving pregnancy outcomes.

Women planning or undergoing pregnancy: Empowered with information, women can actively participate in their care, make informed decisions, and better understand the implications of early interventions.

This book is a call to action – to adopt a proactive, not reactive, stance in maternal healthcare. It aims to promote safer pregnancies, healthier babies, and more informed parents, through a scientifically sound and clinically practical roadmap.

CHAPTER I: THE EVOLUTION OF ANTENATAL CARE

"The journey of antenatal care (ANC) is a reflection of a humanity's evolving understanding of pregnancy, childbirth, and maternal wellbeing."

(A) Ancient Beginnings: Care Rooted in Tradition

The journey of antenatal care (ANC) is a reflection of a humanity's evolving understanding of pregnancy, childbirth, and maternal wellbeing. From ancient rituals to advanced, evidence-based practices, the story of ANC is rich and informative.

Cultural Perceptions and Secrecy

In many cultures, early pregnancy was kept secret due to social taboos, fear of miscarriage, or the belief that early disclosure might bring misfortune. As a result, women often delayed seeking care until the pregnancy was visibly advanced. This contributed to a late-term approach to antenatal check-ups.

The Middle Ages: Midwifery and Mysticism

During the medieval period, antenatal care was informal and largely in **the hands of experienced but scientifically untrained midwives.** Childbirth was considered a natural, a dangerous event. Knowledge was passed orally, and many practices were governed by superstition and religious beliefs. While some midwives possessed impressive empirical knowledge, **the lack of scientific understanding and sterile techniques** led **to high maternal and infant mortality.**

18th and 19th Century: Medicalization of Pregnancy

The industrial age brought significant changes. Medicine became more scientific, and obstetric began to emerge as a distinct field. Hospitals began offering care to pregnant women, particularly those with complications. However, **the care was more curative than preventive.** The rise of puerperal fever led to the adoption of hygiene and antiseptic methods, pioneered by figures like **Ignas Semmelweis** *(was a **Hungarian Physician and Scientist** who was an early pioneer of antiseptic procedures and was described as "saviour of mothers").*

Despite the progress, antenatal care was still fragmented, often inaccessible to rural and poor population. It was in this era that the foundations for modern obstetric practice were laid.

Early 20th Century: The Birth of Structured Antenatal Care

The early 1900[s] marked a turning point. In 1901, **Dr. John William Ballantyne of Edinburgh** introduced the concept of dedicated antenatal clinics. For **the first time** pregnancy care was framed as **preventive and not just reactive.** Clinics began offering regular check-ups, nutritional advice, and screening for common complications like anemia and preeclampsia.

This era recognized the critical **link between maternal and fetal health,** and nations began integrating antenatal care into public health frameworks. Education for expected mothers became an essential component of care.

Post-War Public Health Expansion

Following World War II, antenatal care services expanded rapidly across the globe, particularly in developed nations. Governments and international organizations began investing in maternal and child health programs. **Standardized protocols were developed** to reduce maternal and neonatal mortality.

The period saw the introduction of **tetanus toxoid vaccination**, **iron-folic acid supplementation**, and emphasis on **skilled birth attendants**. The focus broadened to include emotional and social support during pregnancy.

Late 20th Century: Evidence-Based Guidelines and Global Access

In 2002, the World Health Organization **(WHO)** introduced the *Focused Antenatal Care* **(FANC)** model, **recommending four targeted visits** designed to identify risks and provide timely interventions improve outcomes for both mother and baby.

Technological advancements such as **ultrasound, blood testing, and fetal monitoring** were integrated into routine care. Antenatal care became multidisciplinary, involving nutritionists, social workers, and mental health professionals.

21st Century and Beyond: Personalized, Inclusive, and Digital

Modern antenatal care emphasizes **personalization, inclusivity, and accessibility.** There is growing awareness of the role of social determinants, gender dynamics, and mental health in pregnancy outcomes. Telehealth and mobile applications now support remote monitoring, education, and consultation – especially vital in remote or underserved areas.

The future of ANC is one **of holistic, respectful, and evidence-driven care.** It recognizes that supporting a woman during pregnancy is not just about preventing disease – it's about **empowering her with knowledge, dignity and choice**.

(B) Traditional Approach to ANC

Historically, antenatal care was not always a continuous, structured process as seen in modern medicine systems. In many traditional societies, care for pregnant women was primarily reserved for the later stages of pregnancy., often starting only in the third trimester or when physical signs of pregnancy were obvious. This practice reflected both cultural beliefs and practical limitations.

Ancient and Traditional Practices

- **Ancient Egypt, India, and China:** Pregnant women received herbal remedies, spiritual guidance, and dietary advice.

- **Ayurveda:** Texts like Charaka Samhita and Sushruta Samhita discussed pregnancy care, including garbhini paricharya (antenatal regimen).

- Emphasis was mostly on maternal nutrition, rest, and rituals to ensure a healthy baby.

Role of Traditional Birth Attendants

In rural and tribal settings, dais (traditional birth attendants) or elder women in the community were the primary caregivers. Their involvement typically increased closer to the expected date of delivery. Care would involve:

- Observation of fetal movements and abdominal size.

- Herbal tonics to ease labor.

- Dietary restrictions and enhancements.

- Rituals to protect the mother and unborn child.

However, these late-stage interactions, though culturally significant, lacked early screening for complications like anemia, hypertension, or fetal anomalies.

Minimal Early Intervention

Without early antenatal visits, many preventable conditions went undiagnosed:

- Hypertensive disorders of pregnancy

- Gestational diabetes

- Fetal growth restriction

- Infections like syphilis or urinary tract infections

This delayed care model contributed to high maternal and perinatal mortality rates in premodern or underserved settings.

Third Trimester as the Focal Point

In traditional systems, the third trimester was often seen as the true phase of "preparation":

- Rituals for safe delivery (e.g., baby showers or "seemantha" in Indian culture).

- Advice on resting, minimizing physical activity.

- Application of herbal oils.

- Arrangements for home birth.

While these practices provided emotional and social support, they lacked the preventive, diagnostic, and therapeutic scope of modern ANC.

Shifting from Late-Term to Life-Cycle Care

Modern antenatal care recognizes that the foundation of a healthy pregnancy is lead even before conception. The traditional trend of late-term care is now seen as insufficient and potentially hazardous. The shift towards early and frequent check-ups aims to:

- Detect complications early.

- Educate and empower women.

- Promote birth preparedness and complication readiness.

- Integrate maternal care into a continuum of reproductive health services.

(C)Reducing Congenital Birth Defects through Preconception and Early Pregnancy Care

➤ Introduction

Traditional models of antenatal care have long emphasized regular check-ups distributed evenly or **concentrated more in the third trimester**. However emerging research and global health priorities suggest a radical rethinking of this approach. **This new paradigm** is best visualized through **the Inverted Pyramid of Antenatal Care.**

What is the Inverted Pyramid???

The inverted pyramid of antenatal care symbolizes a strategic shift: **it places maximum emphasis on early pregnancy care** – particularly the **first trimester** – as the most critical window for optimizing maternal and fetal outcomes.

In this model:

- The base **(widest part)** of the pyramid **is at the top**, representing intensive care **early in pregnancy.**

- The **narrow tip at the bottom** represents relatively **fewer interventions** needed later, **assuming early care was comprehensive and effective.**

Congenital anomalies—or birth defects—pose a significant global health burden. Worldwide, approximately **2–3% of all live births** are affected by congenital anomalies, with **India reporting a prevalence of 1–3%**. These anomalies range from minor structural issues to severe, life-limiting disorders. Some are compatible with life and long-term functionality, while others result in perinatal mortality or lifelong disability.

With advances in medicine and public health, much of the focus has now shifted from merely treating these conditions to

preventing them through early interventions. This chapter explores the critical role that **preconceptional planning and first trimester antenatal care** can play in significantly reducing the burden of congenital defects.

➢ Understanding Congenital Defects: Magnitude and Impact

Congenital anomalies include structural, functional, or metabolic disorders that develop in utero and are present at birth. Common examples include neural tube defects, congenital heart defects, limb anomalies, cleft lip/palate, and chromosomal abnormalities such as Down syndrome.

- **Global burden**: Approximately 240,000 newborns die worldwide within 28 days of birth due to congenital anomalies.
- **Indian context**: With over 25 million births annually, even a 1% rate equates to **over 2.5 lakh newborns** affected each year in India alone.

These defects not only lead to emotional and financial distress for families but also impose a heavy load on national healthcare systems.

➢ Root Causes and Risk Factors

Congenital anomalies can be attributed to **genetic, environmental, nutritional, and infectious factors**, often with a multifactorial origin.

Key risk factors include:

- **Advanced maternal age**
- **Consanguinity**
- **Nutritional deficiencies (especially folic acid and iodine)**

- **Uncontrolled maternal diseases (e.g., diabetes, epilepsy)**
- **Teratogenic medications**
- **Exposure to infections (e.g., rubella, cytomegalovirus)**
- **Environmental toxins**
- **Alcohol, tobacco, and substance abuse**

> ## The Preventive Power of Preconceptional and Early Pregnancy Care

Early antenatal care, particularly **prior to conception and during the first trimester**, represents a **critical window** to minimize the risk of congenital disorders. Here's how:

1. Preconception Counseling and Risk Assessment

- Encourages **planned pregnancies**, avoiding unintentional exposures during **organogenesis.**
- Identifies couples at higher risk due to genetic history or previous adverse outcomes.
- Enables lifestyle changes (e.g., cessation of alcohol or smoking) before pregnancy begins.

2. Folic Acid Supplementation

- **400 mcg daily** folic acid taken at least **1 month before conception** and continued through the first trimester can reduce **neural tube defects by up to 70%**.

3. Optimizing Maternal Health

- Pre-pregnancy management of **chronic conditions** like diabetes, hypertension, and hypothyroidism ensures a safer intrauterine environment.
- Review of current medications to avoid teratogenic drugs.

4. Screening for Infections and Immunization

- **Rubella and varicella immunity** testing and vaccination before conception.
- Screening for **STIs, HIV, and Hepatitis B/C**, with appropriate treatment and planning.

5. Genetic Counseling and Carrier Screening

- For high-risk couples (e.g., family history, consanguinity, advanced age).
- Can help in informed reproductive decision-making, including IVF with PGD (Preimplantation Genetic Diagnosis) when appropriate.

6. Environmental and Occupational Risk Assessment

- Advising on avoidance of radiation, heavy metals, pesticides, and other known teratogens.

➢ First Trimester Interventions

- **Early ultrasound** helps confirm viability, gestational age, and detect gross anomalies.
- **First-trimester combined screening** (nuchal translucency + serum markers) can identify chromosomal anomalies early.
- **Non-Invasive Prenatal Testing (NIPT)** from 10 weeks onward can detect trisomies with high accuracy.
- Starting iron, omega 3 fatty acids, and iodine supplementation supports optimal fetal development.

➢ **Empowering Couples with Knowledge**

One of the most powerful tools in reducing congenital defects is **education and awareness**. Couples who understand the value of early care are more likely to:

- Seek preconception advice
- Begin folic acid early
- Avoid harmful exposures
- Attend timely antenatal visits

A **proactive health-seeking behavior** can thus shift the curve from reactive treatment to **preventive well-being**.

Conclusion: A Collective Responsibility

Preventing congenital anomalies is not solely the responsibility of the healthcare provider or the mother. It requires **public health policy**, **community education**, **accessible healthcare**, and **individual awareness**. By integrating **preconceptional counseling and first trimester care** into mainstream antenatal practices, we can make a tangible difference in reducing the burden of congenital defects.

Planned pregnancies, timely screening, nutritional optimization, and lifestyle modifications—all play a role in this **silent revolution in maternal and child health**. The road to a healthier next generation begins even before conception.

(D)The Crucial Role of Preconception and Early Antenatal Screening – A case of Thalassemia

"Early screening in first trimester / preconceptional

counselling can prevent lifelong sufferings"

-Anonymous

➢ Introduction

Thalassemia is more than a medical condition – it is a public health concern that brings into sharp focus the essential role of preconceptional counseling and early antenatal screening. Despite its preventability, thousands of children in India are born each year with Thalassemia major, beginning the lifelong battle with chronic illness. This chapter explores how a single, avoidable genetic condition can underscore the necessity of early maternal care.

➢ Genetic Basis: Why Early Identification is Key

Thalassemia is inherited in an **autosomal recessive pattern.**

Beta Thalassemia trait is also known as Beta Thalassemia minor. Normally, beta Thalassemia trait does not cause any major health problem except mild to moderate anaemia. Beta Thalassemia trait is inherited from one's parents. When one parent has beta Thalassemia trait and the other parent has normal haemoglobin A, there are possible outcomes with each pregnancy as follows:

- 50% chance of having a child with beta Thalassemia trait.

- 50% chance of having a child without trait (normal child).

When both parents are carriers (Thalassemia minor), there are possible outcomes with each pregnancy as follows:

- 25% chance of being affected with Thalassemia major

- 50% chances of being a carrier (Thalassemia minor)

- 25% chances of being completely unaffected.

This predictable inheritance pattern makes genetic counseling before conception or in the first trimester absolutely vital.

➢ **Thalassemia in India: A Public Health Perspective**

- India sees approximately 10000 – 12000 births annually of children with Thalassemia major.

- Over 42 million carriers reside in India.

- High-risk communities include Sindhis, Punjabis, Gujaratis, Bengalis, Jains, and some tribal populations.

➢ **Treatment Burden: Blood, Infrastructure, and Lives**

- Children with Thalassemia major require 6 – 16 transfusions annually (often monthly or bimonthly).

- During the COVID-19 pandemic, severe blood shortages were reported across India, especially in rural districts.

- Even in normal times, rural blood banks often face:
  o Inconsistent supply
  o Lack of refrigeration or screening facilities
  o Staffing shortages

➢ **Life Expectancy and Emotional Toll**

- With optimal care (regular transfusions and iron chelation), life expectancy may extend into the third or fourth decade.

- Without access to care, survival may be limited to early adolescence.

- Families often experience:
    o Financial strain
    o Chronic stress and burnout
    o Depression and anxiety linked to watching their child's suffering.

- Bone marrow transplants are a potential cure for Thalassemia major. But the success rate can vary depending on the factors – finding a suitable donor who is a good match for the patient's human leucocyte antigens (HLA), also bone marrow transplants can have potential risks, including graft-versus-host disease (GVHD), infections, and other complications. The cost of bone marrow transplant can range from 8 lakhs to 40 lakhs in India. *(Underprivileged children with Thalassemia and aplastic anemia may be eligible for free bone marrow transplant under the **Central Government's Thalassemia and Aplastic Anemia Bal Seva Yojna.**)*

➢ **Preventive Strategies: A Multi-Tiered Approach**

1. Preconceptional Counseling

- Carrier screening for couples planning a pregnancy.

- Educating at-risk communities about genetic inheritance.

- Preventing carrier-carrier marriages or providing reproductive options.

2. First-Trimester Screening

- Hemoglobin electrophoresis or HPLC to detect carriers.

- Prenatal diagnosis via chorionic villus sampling (CVS) at 10 -12 weeks or amniocentesis at $16 - 18$ weeks.

- Early decision-making, including medical termination, if necessary.

3. Preimplantation Genetic Diagnosis (PGD)

- IVF with genetic testing of embryos can help carrier couples have unaffected children.

- Available in India, though still limited by cost and access.

4. School and Community-Level Screening

- Routine screening in schools, colleges, and marriage bureaus in endemic areas.

- Counseling of young carriers and their families about partner choices.

5. Awareness Campaigns and Policy Integration

- Public health campaigns to normalize carrier status.

- Integration of Thalassemia screening into reproductive health services.

*In summary, this example of Thalassemia major illustrates the high cost of missed opportunities in antenatal care. **Early screening in first trimester / preconceptional counseling can prevent lifelong suffering,** ease the emotional and financial burden on families, and reduce pressure on India's overstretched healthcare infrastructure.*

- ## Premarital Screening:

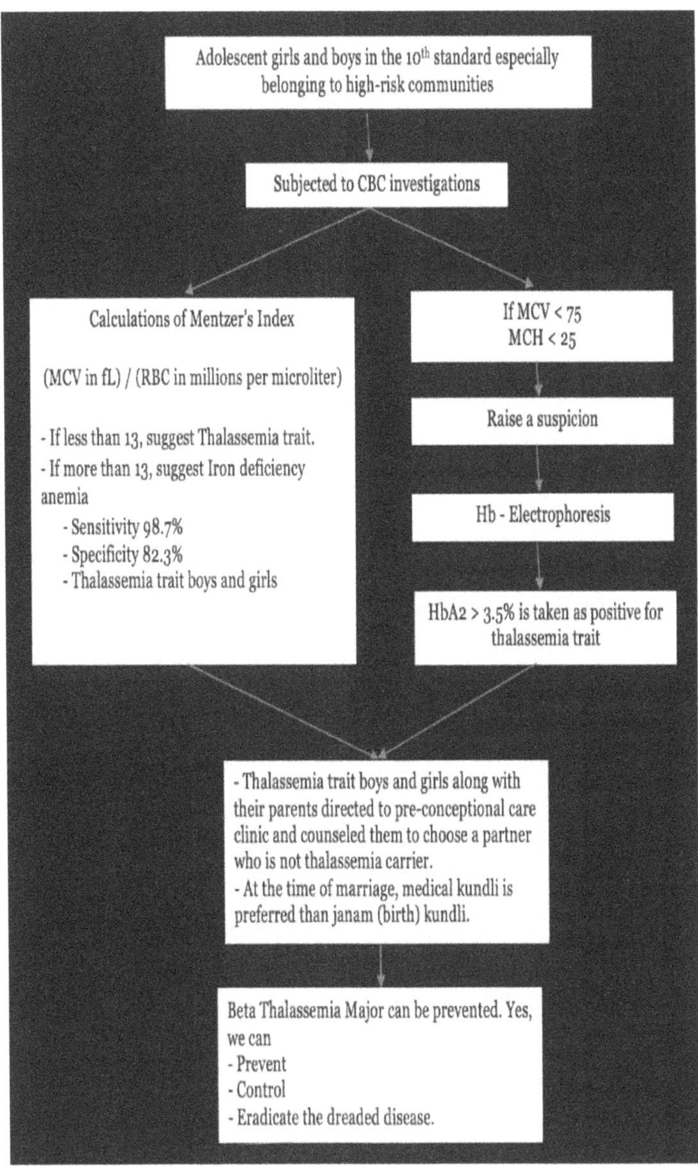

- ## Post-marital Screening:

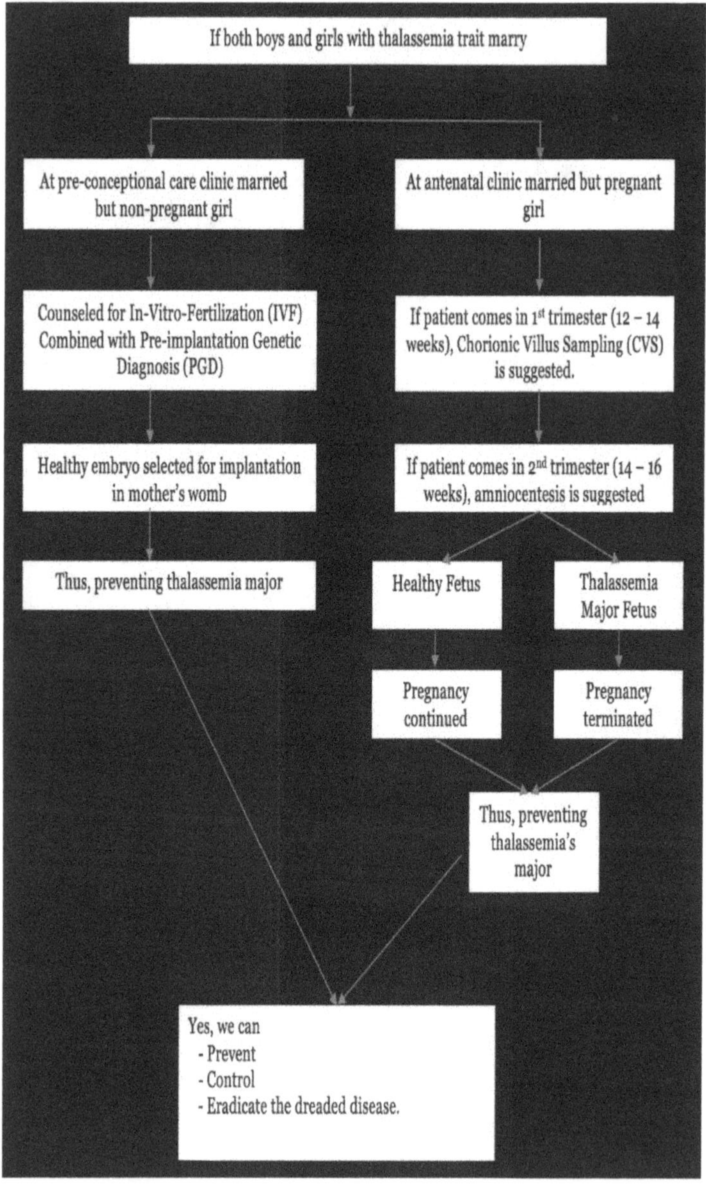

CHAPTER II: PRECONCEPTIONAL COUNSELING

"Before you grow the baby, grow the soil.

Preconception is the time to prepare

a garden of motherhood."

-Anonymous

(A) Importance of Preconceptional Care/Visit

➤ **Introduction**

- o **Definition**: Preconceptional care refers to medical, lifestyle, and psychosocial interventions provided to women (and couples) before conception occurs.

- o **Objective**: To optimize maternal health, identify risks, and create the best possible environment for conception, fetal development, and pregnancy outcomes.

➤ **Why Preconceptional Care Matters**

- o **Major fetal organs develop in the first 8–10 weeks**, often before a woman knows she is pregnant, especially in a woman with irregular cycles.

- o **Lifestyle changes, folic acid supplementation, and chronic disease management** are most effective when started **before conception**.

- o **Preventable adverse outcomes** like neural tube defects, miscarriage, preterm birth, and congenital anomalies can be significantly reduced.

➢ Epidemiological Evidence

- o Studies (e.g., **CDC, WHO**) show:
  - ▪ Nearly **50% of pregnancies are unplanned**, leading to missed opportunities for early care.

  - ▪ Women with **diabetes**, **thyroid disease**, or **hypertension** benefit greatly from early risk management.

  - ▪ Preconception folic acid reduces neural tube defects by **up to 70%**.

➢ Involving the Male Partner

- o Sperm quality is affected by **obesity, smoking, alcohol, and occupational exposures**.

- o Men also benefit from health screenings and lifestyle changes.

- o Promotes shared responsibility and support.

➢ The Public Health Perspective

- o Preconception care is cost-effective and scalable.

- o Reduces maternal morbidity, NICU admissions, and long-term developmental delays.

- o Encouraged by **WHO**, **FIGO**, and other global health organizations.

➢ **Challenges in Implementation**

- o Lack of awareness—most women do not seek care until pregnancy is established.

- o Limited availability of structured preconception clinics.

- o Misconception that the antenatal care begins only after a missed period or ultrasound diagnosis.

➢ **Moving Towards a Proactive Model**

- o Family physicians, OB-GYNs, and community health workers should:
  - **Incorporate preconception discussions** into routine visits.

  - Use **checklists and screening tools** for every woman of reproductive age.

  - Normalize preconception health like annual dental or vision checks.

➢ **Components of Preconceptional Counseling**

After understanding why preconceptional care is a critical foundation for maternal and fetal well-being, it is essential to explore **what this care actually involves**. Preconceptional counseling is not a *one-size-fits-all* approach—it is a **comprehensive, individualized process** aimed at optimizing the health of both partners before pregnancy begins.

The core components of effective preconceptional counseling include:

1. **Identification and management of existing chronic conditions**
2. **Nutritional assessment and lifestyle modifications**
3. **Genetic counseling and family history evaluation**
4. **Vaccination and infection screening**
5. **Medication review and risk factor modification**
6. **Supportive counseling and shared decision-making**

Each of these components contributes to **risk reduction, early intervention, and informed planning**—empowering couples to begin their pregnancy journey with confidence and care.

In the sections that follow, we will explore each of these pillars in detail, with practical insights, current evidence, and patient-centered strategies that make preconceptional care truly impactful.

(B) Identifying and Managing Chronic Conditions

"The first gift you give your child

is a healthy womb.

That gift is wrapped in the months

before conception"

-Anonymous

➢ **Introduction**

- o Chronic conditions like **diabetes, hypertension, thyroid dysfunction, epilepsy, obesity**, and **autoimmune disorders** can significantly impact fertility, fetal development, and maternal well-being.

- o Early identification and optimization **before conception** improves maternal outcomes and reduces risk of miscarriage, fetal anomalies, and growth restrictions.

➢ **Systematic Approach to Preconception Screening**

- o **Medical History**
  - Detailed personal and family history

  - Menstrual and reproductive history (infertility, miscarriages, ectopic)

  - Past obstetric complications (e.g., preeclampsia, IUGR, GDM)

- o **Physical Examination**
  - BMI, blood pressure, thyroid gland, signs of insulin resistance or anemia

- o **Baseline Investigations**
  - CBC, Blood group Rh, VDRL, HBsAg, HIV, FBS/HbA1c, TSH, Renal and Liver profile, Vitamin D, urine (routine, micro).

  - Additional tests: ANA, APLA, HCV, not mandatory but required depending on history.

- o **Chronic Conditions: Identification and Preconception Management**
  - **Diabetes Mellitus (Type 1/Type 2)**
    - ✓ Optimize HbA1c to **<6.5%** before conception.
    - ✓ Avoid conception during poor glycemic control.
    - ✓ Transition to **pregnancy-safe medications** (e.g., insulin).
    - ✓ Screening for nephropathy, retinopathy, and cardiovascular risks.

  - **Hypertension**
    - ✓ Discontinue teratogenic drugs (e.g., ACE inhibitors, ARBs).
    - ✓ Switch to safer options like **labetalol, nifedipine, methyldopa.**
    - ✓ Check for end-organ damage (renal, cardiac).

  - **Hypothyroidism**
    - ✓ Maintain **TSH <2.5 mIU/L** before conception.
    - ✓ Adjust levothyroxine dosage based on TSH.
    - ✓ Autoimmune screening (Anti-TPO) if relevant.

- **Epilepsy**
  - ✓ Detailed review of seizure history and control.
  - ✓ Switch from valproate (high risk of congenital malformations) to safer AEDs like **lamotrigine** or **carbamazepine.**
  - ✓ Start **high-dose folic acid (4–5 mg/day)**

- **Obesity & PCOS**
  - ✓ Encourage **weight loss** before conception (5–10% weight loss can restore ovulation).
  - ✓ Address insulin resistance (metformin use, if applicable).
  - ✓ Counsel on risks of miscarriage, GDM, macrosomia.

- **Autoimmune Disorders (e.g., SLE, RA)**
  - ✓ Plan conception during **disease remission**
  - ✓ Evaluate medications: some **DMARDs** *(Disease modifying antirheumatic Drugs)* are contraindicated.
  - ✓ Risk of flare, thrombosis, and fetal loss must be discussed.

- **Renal or Hepatic Disorders**
  - ✓ Assess baseline function
  - ✓ Discuss potential pregnancy complications (e.g., preeclampsia, IUGR)
  - ✓ Involve multidisciplinary care team early.

➢ **Multidisciplinary Coordination**

- o Involve endocrinologists, neurologists, nephrologists, or rheumatologists as needed.

- o A team approach ensures comprehensive care and risk mitigation.

- **Case Study Box: "The Missed Window"**

  - A 28-year-old woman B with poorly controlled Type 2 diabetes conceives. She presents at 10 weeks with HbA1c of 9%. Despite best efforts, her baby is diagnosed with congenital heart defect.
  - Whereas another woman C who optimized diabetes control preconceptionally had a healthy outcome.

- **Counseling and Empowerment**

  - Discuss long-term benefits of early optimization—not only for pregnancy but for future maternal health.
  - Encourage active patient participation in managing their condition.

Summary Chart: Chronic Condition → Preconception Goal → Action Plan

Condition	Goal Before Conception	Action
Diabetes	HbA1c <6.5%	Lifestyle + insulin adjustment
Hypothyroidism	TSH <2.5 mIU/L	Adjust thyroxine dose
Hypertension	Normotension on safe meds	Switch to labetalol, methyldopa
Epilepsy	Seizure control + safe AED	Avoid valproate; add folic acid
Obesity	BMI around 30	Weight loss, diet, exercise
Autoimmune	Remission state	Adjust medicines, multidisciplinary care

(C) Nutritional Advice and Lifestyle Modifications

"When we shift care to the beginning,

we protect everything that follows"

-Anonymous

➢ **Introduction**

- o Nutrition and lifestyle are **modifiable risk factors** that strongly influence fertility, conception success, fetal organogenesis, and long-term child health (Developmental Origins of Health and Disease – DOHaD).

- o Preconception is the **ideal time** to correct deficiencies, normalize weight, and eliminate habits that harm maternal-fetal outcomes.

➢ **Preconception Nutritional Assessment**

- o **BMI & Body Composition**
  Aim for BMI between **18.5 and 24.9** for optimal fertility and pregnancy outcomes.

- o **Dietary History**
  Look for trends in fast food, irregular meals, nutrient-poor diets, vegetarianism/veganism without supplements.

- o **Screening for Deficiencies**
  Iron, folate, Vitamin B12, D3, calcium, iodine, omega-3 fatty acids.

➢ **Balanced Preconception Diet Plan**

o **Macro Balance**: Complex carbs, lean protein, healthy fats.
o **Micros**: Fruits, vegetables, whole grains, nuts/seeds, legumes.
o **Hydration**: 8–10 glasses/day.

o **Avoid**:
  ▪ Processed foods, excess caffeine (>200 mg/day), sugar-rich beverages, and trans fats.
  ▪ Detox or keto diets that impair fertility.

➢ **Key Nutrients and Preconception Recommendations**

Nutrient	Why It's Important	Dosage / Advice
Folic Acid	Prevents neural tube defects	**400–800 mcg/day**, start **at least 1 month** before conception
Iron	Prevents anemia, supports placental growth	27–30 mg/day (or as per Hb level)
Vitamin D	Supports immune and bone health	600–1000 IU/day or as per serum levels
Calcium	Essential for fetal bones, maternal reserves	1000–1200 mg/day
Iodine	Prevents cretinism, supports thyroid function	150 mcg/day (through iodized salt/supplement)
Omega-3 (DHA/EPA)	Brain and retinal development	200–300 mg/day
Vitamin B12	Prevents anemia and neural defects (esp. in vegetarians)	2.4 mcg/day or supplements

- ➢ **Lifestyle Modifications**

  - ○ **Weight Management**

    - ▪ Obesity increases risks for GDM, preeclampsia, miscarriage, stillbirth.

    - ▪ Underweight increases risk for LBW and preterm birth.

    - ▪ **Target: 5–10% weight loss for overweight women** before conceiving.

  - ○ **Exercise**

    - ▪ Encourage **moderate-intensity activity**: 30 minutes, 5 times/week (e.g., brisk walking, yoga, swimming).

    - ▪ Improves ovulatory function, insulin sensitivity, and mental health.

  - ○ **Sleep Hygiene**

    - ▪ 7–9 hours of restful sleep per night.

    - ▪ Poor sleep linked with hormonal imbalances and metabolic syndrome.

  - ○ **Stress Management**

    - ▪ High stress disrupts ovulation, increases cortisol and inflammation.

    - ▪ Include:
      Yoga, meditation, journaling, therapy if needed.

- o **Avoiding Harmful Substances**

Substance	Risks
Smoking (including passive)	IUGR, miscarriage, ectopic, placental issues
Alcohol	Fetal alcohol spectrum Disorder
Recreational drugs	Teratogenicity, poor neurodevelopment
Caffeine	>200 mg/day linked to Miscarriage

- o **Partner's Lifestyle Matters Too**

  - ▪ Smoking, alcohol, obesity, and poor diet can impair **sperm DNA integrity**.

  - ▪ Counsel couples together, when possible, for shared accountability.

- ➢ **Summary Box: Quick Preconception Lifestyle Checklist**

Lifestyle Factor	Goal
BMI	18.5–24.9
Folic Acid	≥400 mcg/day
Iron & Vitamin D	Correct deficiencies
Exercise	150 min/week
Caffeine	<200 mg/day
Tobacco/Alcohol/Drugs	Stop completely
Stress & Sleep	Manage and optimize

- ➢ **Why Folic Acid Prescription at 2 Months (8 Weeks) is Too Late for Preventing Neural Tube Defects (NTDs)???**
  - **Key Fact:**
    - o The **neural tube closes by Day 28 post-conception** (around **6 weeks of gestation**, counting from LMP).

    - o By the time most women present at 8 weeks (2 months), **the critical window for preventing NTDs is already passed**.

"Starting folic acid at 8 weeks is like closing the door after the horse has bolted. The neural tube has already closed."

  - **Timeline of Neural Tube Development:**

Event	Gestational Age
Fertilization	~Week 2
Neural Plate formation	Week 3
Neural Tube closure	Between **Day 21–28** (Week 4–6 of gestation)

*So, **folic acid must be present in adequate levels during the periconceptional period (1 month before and first month after conception)** to be effective in preventing NTDs like spina bifida and anencephaly.*

Then Why Do Doctors Still Prescribe Folic Acid if Patient Comes After 2 Months?

While it's **too late to prevent neural tube defects**, folic acid may still offer other benefits:

- **Supports placental development.**

- **Reduces risk of anemia** in the mother.

- May help in **preventing other congenital abnormalities**, though evidence is weaker than for NTDs.

- It's part of **standard antenatal supplements** (with iron, calcium, etc.).

- But for **NTD prevention**, it's **ineffective if started after the 6th gestational week**.

Implications for Clinical Practice:

- **All women of reproductive age** who might become pregnant should be on folic acid **before they even conceive**.

- Preconception counseling should include **400–800 mcg/day of folic acid**, increased to **4–5 mg/day** for high-risk cases (e.g., prior NTD, epilepsy, diabetes).

- This underscores the need to **shift antenatal care to the preconception and first-trimester stage—**

(D) Genetic Counseling and Family History

"A well-informed mother is the best

foundation for a healthy generation"

-Anonymous

➢ **Introduction**

- o Genetic counseling aims to assess the **risk of inherited conditions** in a pregnancy and guide families in understanding the implications, testing options, and reproductive decisions.

- o Preconception is the **ideal time** to do this—**before conception**, when couples have **time, choices, and clarity.**

➢ **Importance of Genetic Evaluation Before Pregnancy**

- o **Allows timely decision-making**: Screening, further testing, or IVF with PGD (preimplantation genetic diagnosis).

- o **Reduces anxiety** and helps in **informed consent** for future interventions.

- o **Identifies risk factors** that may otherwise remain hidden until anomalies arise during pregnancy.

➢ **Detailed Family History: A Key Screening Tool**

- o A **3-generation pedigree** should be taken for:

  - ▪ Birth defects, intellectual disability, developmental delay.

- Genetic syndromes (e.g., thalassemia, Tay-Sachs, cystic fibrosis, muscular dystrophy)

- Recurrent miscarriages, stillbirths, infertility.

- Consanguinity.

- Ethnicity-linked conditions (e.g., sickle cell in African ancestry, thalassemia in South Asians).

➢ **Sample Checklist:**

Family History Element Screening Suggestion

Family History Element	Screening Suggestion
Sibling with thalassemia	Do HPLC of both partners
History of Down syndrome	Offer karyotyping or NIPT counseling
Recurrent miscarriages	Screen for antiphospholipid syndrome & chromosomal translocations
Parental consanguinity	Offer broader carrier screening panel
Intellectual disability in family	Consider Fragile X testing

➢ **When to Refer for Genetic Counseling**

You should **refer the couple to a genetic counselor** or geneticist if:

- ✓ Either parent is a **known carrier** of a genetic disorder.
- ✓ There is a **previous child with congenital anomalies.**
- ✓ There is a **history of multiple pregnancy losses.**
- ✓ **Advanced maternal age** ($\geq$35 years).

✓ **Consanguinity.**
✓ One partner has a **chronic disease with teratogenic treatment** (e.g., epilepsy, cancer).

➢ **Carrier Screening**

Targeted carrier screening based on ethnic background or history:

✓ Thalassemia
✓ Sickle cell disease
✓ Spinal Muscular Atrophy (SMA)
✓ Fragile X syndrome
✓ Cystic Fibrosis (in Western populations)

Expanded carrier panels available via blood or saliva, especially in IVF clinics.

➢ **Counseling for High-Risk Couples**

If both partners are carriers of an autosomal recessive condition (e.g., thalassemia minor):

- There is a **25% chance** of an affected child with thalassemia major.
  - Options include:
    - ✓ IVF + Preimplantation Genetic Diagnosis (PGD)
    - ✓ Early prenatal diagnosis via CVS/Amniocentesis
    - ✓ Counseling about outcomes and decisions

- **Patient Communication Tips**
  - Use **simple, non-technical language** to explain risk percentages.
  - Emphasize that "being a carrier is not a disease" but planning is important.

- o Provide **written summaries** and offer a follow-up session if needed.
- o Avoid alarmist tone—focus on empowerment and informed choice.

➢ **Real-Life Example Box:**

*A couple with no symptoms is found to be thalassemia minor carriers during preconception workup. They had no idea of the risk. Genetic counseling guided them to opt for PGD and they **had a healthy child free of the disease.** **Contrast:** A similar couple found out only during second trimester, and **had to make a difficult decision**.*

➢ **Summary Box: Take-Home Messages**

Key Insight	Clinical Implication
Family history reveals hidden risks	Take a 3-generation pedigree
Carrier screening is now accessible	Offer it based on history or ethnicity
Early referral allows wider choices	IVF with PGD or early prenatal testing
Empower, don't alarm	Use calm and clear language

➢ **Preconception Family History Questionnaire**

- **Section A: Couple Information**
  - o **Age of female partner**: _______
  - o **Age of male partner**: _______
  - o **Are you related by blood (consanguinity)?** Yes / No
    If yes, specify relation: _________________

- **Section B: Personal & Reproductive History**
  - o Have you had:

- Recurrent miscarriages (≥2)
- Stillbirth or neonatal death
- Infertility or subfertility
- Previous child with birth defect or genetic condition

o Do either of you have:
  - Intellectual disability or developmental delay
  - Vision or hearing loss from birth
  - Seizure disorder or neurologic disease
  - Congenital heart defect
  - Physical deformity or dysmorphic features

- **Section C: Family History (3 Generations)**

For each condition below, tick if present in:

Condition	You	Partner	Family (mention relation)
Thalassemia	[ ]	[ ]	_________________
Sickle Cell Anemia	[ ]	[ ]	_________________
Down Syndrome or chromosomal disorder	[ ]	[ ]	_________________
Muscular Dystrophy	[ ]	[ ]	_________________
Spinal Muscular Atrophy (SMA)	[ ]	[ ]	_________________
Fragile X Syndrome	[ ]	[ ]	_________________
Cystic Fibrosis	[ ]	[ ]	_________________
Hemophilia / Bleeding disorder	[ ]	[ ]	_________________
Autism / developmental delay	[ ]	[ ]	_________________
Deafness / blindness from childhood	[ ]	[ ]	_________________
Metabolic diseases (e.g., PKU)	[ ]	[ ]	_________________
Others (specify): ________________	[ ]	[ ]	_________________

- **Section D: Ethnic / Regional Background**
  - o Are you or your partner from a community with high prevalence of any specific condition (e.g., Sindhi, Punjabi, Gujarati, Tribal groups)?
  If yes, please specify: _______________________

  - o Have you undergone any previous genetic or carrier screening?
  If yes, share reports if available.

➢ **Common Inherited Disorders: Global and Indian Context**

A variety of inherited disorders may affect couples planning pregnancy. Some are more common globally, while others are region-specific to India. Below is a brief overview presented in a narrative-friendly format.

1) **Thalassemia (Beta-Thalassemia)**
   An autosomal recessive disorder commonly found in India, particularly in Gujarat, Punjab, West Bengal, and Maharashtra. Carrier frequency in these areas may reach up to 10%. All at-risk couples should undergo HPLC or genetic testing prior to conception.

2) **Sickle Cell Anemia**
   Also, autosomal recessive, this condition is prevalent in tribal belts of Odisha, Madhya Pradesh, Chhattisgarh, Maharashtra, and Gujarat. Routine hemoglobin electrophoresis or sickle solubility testing is advised, especially in high-risk ethnic groups.

3) **G6PD Deficiency**
   An X-linked recessive enzymopathy, it is seen across Africa, the Middle East, and parts of India. Though often asymptomatic, it can lead to severe hemolysis in neonates exposed to oxidant drugs or infections.

4) **Down Syndrome**
   Caused by Trisomy 21, this chromosomal disorder has
   no ethnic predisposition but shows strong correlation
   with increasing maternal age. Preconception genetic
   counseling is vital, particularly in women above 35
   years.

5) **Fragile X Syndrome**
   An X-linked dominant disorder, it is the most common
   inherited cause of intellectual disability. While
   globally prevalent, screening is usually reserved for
   individuals with a family history of developmental
   delays, autism, or unexplained intellectual disability.

6) **Cystic Fibrosis**
   This autosomal recessive disorder is widespread in
   Western populations, especially in Europe and the US.
   It remains rare in India but is increasingly detected due
   to awareness and expanded carrier screening.

7) **Spinal Muscular Atrophy (SMA)**
   An autosomal recessive neurodegenerative condition
   with a global footprint. Carrier screening is now part
   of expanded genetic panels, and preimplantation
   diagnosis is available for high-risk couples.

8) **Tay-Sachs Disease**
   Rare in India but common in **Ashkenazi Jewish** and
   French-Canadian populations. Screening is usually
   ethnicity-targeted.

9) **Hemophilia (A and B)**
   X-linked recessive bleeding disorders seen globally. A
   family history in males warrants carrier testing in
   females, especially before invasive procedures or
   conception.

10) **Congenital Deafness**
Caused by multiple genetic factors, often inherited in autosomal recessive fashion. **Consanguinity** significantly increases risk, especially in certain Indian populations. Early genetic counseling and screening are advised.

> **Top 5 Inherited Disorders to Screen for in India**

1) Beta-Thalassemia

- **Why**: High carrier rate in multiple Indian states (Gujarat, Punjab, West Bengal, Maharashtra).
- **Screening**: Hemoglobin electrophoresis or HPLC for both partners.
- **Inheritance**: Autosomal Recessive.
- **Impact**: Major thalassemia requires lifelong transfusions if both partners are carriers.

2) Sickle Cell Anemia

- **Why**: Common in tribal populations across Odisha, MP, Maharashtra, and Gujarat.
- **Screening**: Sickle solubility test, hemoglobin electrophoresis.
- **Inheritance**: Autosomal Recessive.
- **Impact**: Severe anemia, painful crises, and fetal complications if untreated.

3) G6PD Deficiency

- **Why**: Frequently encountered in Indian males; risk of neonatal jaundice and hemolysis.
- **Screening**: Enzyme activity test.
- **Inheritance**: X-linked Recessive.

- **Impact**: Avoidance of oxidant drugs and stressors is essential in affected individuals.

4) Spinal Muscular Atrophy (SMA)

- **Why**: Global prevalence; increasingly included in expanded carrier screening panels in India.
- **Screening**: SMN1 gene deletion testing (blood-based).
- **Inheritance**: Autosomal Recessive.
- **Impact**: Progressive neuromuscular degeneration; severe forms lead to infant death if untreated.

5) Congenital Deafness (Hereditary Sensorineural Hearing Loss)

- **Why**: Common in consanguineous families and certain Indian communities.
- **Screening**: Targeted gene panels or family history-based testing.
- **Inheritance**: Usually Autosomal Recessive.
- **Impact**: Early detection enables timely intervention (e.g., cochlear implants).

*If either partner is from a high-risk region or if there is consanguinity or family history, offer **targeted or expanded genetic screening before conception**.*

> **Expanded Genetic Screening Before Conception in Consanguinity**

Why Is It Needed?

- Consanguineous couples (e.g., first or second cousins) share a higher percentage of genes.

- The chance of both partners carrying the same **recessive pathogenic variant** is much higher.

- Many **rare disorders** that may not be routinely screened in the general population can manifest in consanguineous unions.

➢ **Recommended Expanded Carrier Screening Panel**

These disorders may not be obvious from family history alone and require genetic testing.

Common Autosomal Recessive Conditions to Screen For:

1. **Beta-Thalassemia and Sickle Cell Anemia**
2. **Spinal Muscular Atrophy (SMA)**
3. **Congenital Deafness (GJB2 mutation and others)**
4. **Cystic Fibrosis (CFTR gene mutations)**
5. **Glycogen Storage Disorders (e.g., GSD I, III)**
6. **Lysosomal Storage Disorders** (e.g., Tay-Sachs, Gaucher, MPS)
7. **Maple Syrup Urine Disease (MSUD)**
8. **Phenylketonuria (PKU)**
9. **Congenital Adrenal Hyperplasia (CAH)**
10. **Fanconi Anemia**
11. **Neuronal Ceroid Lipofuscinosis (NCLs)**
12. **Wilson Disease**
13. **Alpha-1 Antitrypsin Deficiency**
14. **Fragile X Syndrome** (X-linked – test for females)
15. **Hemophilia A/B** (if there is family history – test for female carriers)

How Is Screening Done?

- **Method**: Blood or saliva-based DNA testing (NGS panels or targeted mutation panels).
- **Who to Test**:
  o Ideally both partners.
  o Start with **female partner**; if she's a carrier, test the male partner for the same condition.
- **When**: **Before conception** or as early in the first trimester as possible.

What If Both Are Carriers for the Same Disorder?

- **Genetic Counseling**: Discuss risk of disease (25% per pregnancy).
- **Reproductive Options**:
  o In-vitro fertilization (IVF) with **Preimplantation Genetic Diagnosis (PGD)**
  o Prenatal diagnosis: Chorionic villus sampling (CVS) or amniocentesis
  o Use of donor gametes
  o Adoption or opting not to conceive

➢ **Case Example Box**

A consanguineous couple AB with no family history underwent expanded carrier screening. Both were found to be carriers of a rare lysosomal storage disorder. **With IVF and PGD, they were able to have a healthy, unaffected child.**

Ethical and Cultural Sensitivity

- Handle discussions with empathy.
- Respect religious or cultural beliefs about pregnancy termination or assisted reproduction.
- Provide written materials and referrals to clinical geneticists when needed.

(E)Vaccination and Infection Screening Before Conception

This is a vital yet often overlooked area that directly impacts **maternal safety, fetal development**, and **pregnancy outcomes**—especially in countries like India, where immunity status is frequently unknown.

➢ Introduction

- Preconception is the **ideal time** to assess **immunity status** and **screen for infections** that can affect both fertility and fetal development.

- Several infections, if contracted **during early pregnancy**, can lead to miscarriage, congenital anomalies, or long-term health issues in the child.

- Some **live vaccines are contraindicated in pregnancy**, making it essential to **vaccinate beforehand**.

➢ Who Should Be Screened or Vaccinated?

- All women planning pregnancy

- Women with:
  - History of recurrent miscarriage or stillbirth
  - Known high-risk exposure (healthcare workers, food handlers)

- o No documented vaccination history
- o Consanguinity or immunosuppression

➢ **Counseling Tips**
- Emphasize **safety of vaccines** and benefits to baby.

- Provide **written information** to counter vaccine hesitancy.

- For live vaccines (MMR, Varicella), advise **1-month contraception** post-vaccination.

➢ **Key Vaccinations to Access and Update Before Pregnancy**
- **Rubella (German measles)**
  - o Importance: Prevents serious birth defects like heart problems, blindness, and deafness.
  - o Action: Check Rubella IgG. If non-immune, give MMR vaccine. Avoid pregnancy for **at least 1 month** after vaccination.

- **Hepatitis B**
  - o Importance: Prevents maternal liver complications and vertical transmission.
  - o Action: Screen with HBsAg. If negative, start 3-dose vaccination series.

- **Varicella (Chickenpox)**
  - o Importance: Prevents fetal deformities and skin scars from congenital varicella.
  - o Action: Check IgG if no prior infection. If non-immune, vaccinate. Avoid conception for **1 month**.

- **Hepatitis A**
  - o Importance: Prevents viral hepatitis in pregnancy.
  - o Action: Vaccinate pre-pregnancy in endemic areas (India included).

- **HPV Vaccine**
  - o Importance: Protects against cervical cancer and genital warts.
  - o Action: Give before conception, especially in women $\leq$ **26 years**.

- **Tetanus, Diphtheria, and Pertussis (Tdap)**
  - o Importance: Protects newborns from tetanus and whooping cough.
  - o Action: Update if not given in the last 10 years. Can also be given in third trimester.

- **Influenza (Flu Shot)**
  - o Importance: Reduces risk of hospitalization during flu outbreaks.
  - o Action: Can be given before or during pregnancy (especially in flu season).

- **COVID-19 Vaccine**
  - o Importance: Reduces maternal complications from COVID during pregnancy.
  - o Action: Safe and recommended before and during pregnancy.

5)TORCH and Other Infections

- **Toxoplasmosis**
  - o Risk: Miscarriage, brain calcifications, hydrocephalus in fetus.
  - o Action: IgG/IgM testing if high-risk (undercooked meat, cats, rural exposure).

- **Rubella**
  - o Risk: Congenital rubella syndrome – severe anomalies.
  - o Action: IgG testing. If non-immune, vaccinate pre-pregnancy (MMR).

- **Cytomegalovirus (CMV)**
  - o Risk: Hearing loss, neurodevelopmental delay.
  - o Action: Routine screening not advised, but emphasize hygiene precautions.

- **Herpes Simplex Virus (HSV)**
  - o Risk: Preterm labor, neonatal encephalitis if acquired near delivery.
  - o Action: Take sexual history. Consider type-specific IgG testing if concerned.

- **HIV, Hepatitis B & C, Syphilis**
  - o Risk: Stillbirth, IUGR, congenital infection.
  - o Action: Mandatory screening during preconception or early pregnancy. Begin treatment if needed.

➢ **Preconception Vaccine & Infection Checklist**

Screening/Vaccine	Done	Notes
Rubella IgG / MMR vaccine	☐	Live vaccine – avoid pregnancy for 1 month
Hepatitis B Screening & Vaccine	☐	3 doses if negative
Varicella IgG / Vaccine	☐	Live vaccine – avoid pregnancy for 1 month
TORCH Panel	☐	Screen if high-risk
HIV / HBsAg / VDRL	☐	Mandatory in most antenatal setups
COVID-19 Vaccine	☐	Safe and recommended
HPV Vaccine (if ≤26)	☐	Complete schedule before conception

➢ **Case Illustration Box**

*A 28-year-old woman R planning her first pregnancy was found **non-immune to rubella and varicella**. She received both vaccines and waited **a month before conceiving.** Six months later, **a rubella outbreak occurred in her community**—but she was **protected.** Her **baby was born healthy and immune**.*

(F) Medication Review of Existing Diseases and Risk Modifications Before Pregnancy

"Preconception care may be invisible,

but its impact echoes through a lifetime"

-Anonymous

This chapter is especially important because many **chronic conditions require medications** that may not be safe in pregnancy, and some risk factors—when modified early—can significantly improve maternal and fetal outcomes.

- ➤ **Introduction**
  - Many women are on **long-term medications** for conditions like **diabetes, epilepsy, hypertension, thyroid disorders, psychiatric illness**, etc.
  - Some of these drugs are **teratogenic** (can harm the developing baby) and must be **reviewed and modified** before conception.
  - The goal is to balance **disease control** and **fetal safety**.

- ➤ **Principles of Preconception Medication Review**
  - **Stop teratogenic medications**
  - **Substitute with pregnancy-safe alternatives**
  - **Ensure disease is well-controlled** before conception
  - **Use the lowest effective dose**
  - **Add protective supplements** (e.g., high-dose folic acid)

- ➤ **Common Conditions and Medication Modifications**
  - **Epilepsy**
    - **Avoid:** Valproate, phenytoin, phenobarbital (high risk of birth defects).
    - **Prefer: Lamotrigine, Levetiracetam** (safer in pregnancy).

- o **Add: Folic acid 4–5 mg/day** at least 3 months preconception.

- **Hypertension**
  - o **Avoid:** ACE inhibitors (e.g., enalapril), ARBs (e.g., losartan).
  - o **Prefer: Labetalol, Methyldopa, Nifedipine**.
  - o **Check for** target organ damage (renal, retinal).

- **Diabetes Mellitus**
  - o **Avoid:** Oral hypoglycemics with teratogenic potential (e.g., some sulfonylureas).
  - o **Prefer: Insulin or Metformin** (with close monitoring).
  - o **Goal HbA1c:** <6.5% before conception.

- **Hypothyroidism**
  - o **Continue Levothyroxine**, but adjust dose based on TSH.
  - o **Goal:** TSH <2.5 mIU/L before conception.
  - o **Monitor** closely once pregnancy is confirmed.

- **Depression / Anxiety / Psychiatric Illness**
  - o **Avoid:** Lithium (in first trimester), valproate, paroxetine.
  - o **Prefer: Sertraline, Fluoxetine, Quetiapine** (under supervision).
  - o **Involve psychiatrist** in preconception planning.

- **Autoimmune Diseases (e.g., SLE, RA)**
  - o **Avoid:** Methotrexate, Mycophenolate, Cyclophosphamide.
  - o **Prefer: Hydroxychloroquine, Azathioprine, Prednisolone**.
  - o **Plan conception** during **disease remission**.

- **Asthma**
  - o **Inhaled corticosteroids** and bronchodilators are generally safe.

- o **Encourage good control** to avoid hypoxia in early pregnancy.

➢ **Supplementation Add-ons Based on Risk**
  - o **Folic Acid 4–5 mg/day**: For patients with epilepsy, diabetes, obesity, or history of NTDs.
  - o **Calcium & Vitamin D**: For those on corticosteroids or antiepileptics.
  - o **Iron**: If there's anemia or high-risk diet.

➢ **Risk Modifications Before Pregnancy**

Risk Factor	Modification Strategy
Obesity	Weight loss (5–10%), diet, exercise
Smoking, Alcohol, Drugs	Complete cessation preconception
Poorly controlled chronic illness	Optimize control before conceiving
Stress / Sleep issues	Mindfulness, sleep hygiene, counseling
Teratogenic drug use	Substitute or stop at least 3 months before conception

➢ **Red Flags for Medication Review**
  - o Women with chronic illness on long-term treatment
  - o History of miscarriage or fetal anomalies
  - o Self-medication or use of alternative remedies
  - o Planned pregnancy without prior medical consultation

"What works for the mother may harm the baby—reviewing and adjusting medications before pregnancy is one of the most important steps in protecting the unborn child."

(G) Challenges / Obstacles in Preconceptional Care

"Conception is an event.

Preparation is a journey.

Preconception care bridges both."

-Anonymous

1. Lack of Awareness: Many individuals and couples are unaware of the importance of preconception care in improving maternal and fetal outcome.

2. Delayed Healthcare Seeking Behavior: Women often seek care only after conception, missing the opportunity for risk assessment and health optimization.

3. Limited Access to Healthcare Services: Geographic, financial, and systemic barriers can prevent access to preconception counseling and care, especially in rural or underserved areas.

4. Sociocultural Beliefs and Stigma: Cultural norms may discourage discussions around reproductive planning, contraception, and fertility optimization.

5. Inadequate Training of Healthcare Providers: Some providers may lack updated knowledge or protocols to effectively counsel patients in the preconception period.

6. Poor Integration into Routine Healthcare:
Preconceptional care is not always integrated into primary or reproductive health visits, leading to missed opportunities.

7. Unplanned Pregnancies: About 50% of pregnancies are unplanned. A high rate of unplanned pregnancies diminishes the window to intervene before conception.

8. Lifestyle Factors and Behavioral Risks: Tobacco use, alcohol consumption, poor diet, and sedentary lifestyles may not be addressed until pregnancy is confirmed.

9. Chronic Disease Management: Conditions like diabetes, hypertension, thyroid disorders, and obesity are often sub-optimally managed to conception.

10. Mental Health and Psychological Factors: Depression, anxiety, and intimate partner violence are frequently overlooked in the preconception period.

11. Inconsistent Guidelines and Policies: Lack of standardized national or institutional policies may lead to inconsistent practices in preconception care delivery.

12. Limited Male Involvement: Preconception care is often seen as a woman's responsibility, overlooking the role of paternal health in fertility and offspring health.

CHAPTER III: FIRST TRIMESTER: THE CRITICAL WINDOW

(A) Milestones in First Trimester Development

The first trimester is a masterclass in biology. Spanning from **week 1 to week 12**, this is a period of **rapid growth, vulnerability, and foundational development**. Every cell division, hormonal surge, and physiological response plays a pivotal role in setting the course for a healthy pregnancy and baby. Unlike the dramatic changes seen in the third trimester, the first trimester unfolds silently — often before the mother even realizes she is pregnant. Yet, it is during these first twelve weeks that life makes its most complex transitions.

The first trimester is a silent revolution in a woman's body. While externally subtle, internally, **organogenesis — the formation of organs — is in full swing**. This process, which largely occurs between **weeks 3 and 8** (embryonic stage), is exquisitely sensitive to both nutritional support and toxic exposures. In this context, nutrition becomes not just a maternal concern but a **lifelong investment in the health and potential of the unborn child**.

> **Understanding Organogenesis: A Vulnerable Yet Powerful Phase**

Organogenesis begins shortly after implantation (pre-embryonic stage) and continues through the embryonic stage, laying the blueprint for the heart, brain, spine, kidneys, limbs, and more. By the end of **week 8**, most major organs are formed and begin rudimentary functioning.

This is the **most sensitive time to nutritional deficits** or teratogenic exposure. A deficiency during this phase doesn't just delay development — it can cause irreversible structural defects. This is why **nutritional counseling and**

supplementation must begin preconceptionally or as early as possible in pregnancy.

> ➢ **Week-by-Week Developmental Milestones**

Weeks 1–4: Pregnancy technically begins from the first day of the last menstrual period (LMP). Fertilization occurs around week 2, when the sperm meets the egg in the fallopian tube. By week 3, the zygote transforms into a blastocyst and implants itself into the uterine wall. Week 4 marks the formation of the gestational sac and early embryonic disc — the foundation of life has been laid.

Weeks 5–6: The **neural tube** begins to form, which later develops into the **brain and spinal cord**. The tiny heart tube begins to beat around day 22 post-conception — a powerful moment in prenatal development. Limb buds start to appear. Ultrasound may detect a yolk sac and possibly a flicker of cardiac activity.

Weeks 7–8: By now, the embryo is developing facial features — eyes, nostrils, and mouth structures are forming. The beginnings of arms and legs are evident. The brain is rapidly growing, and the digestive tract starts forming. Despite the small size (around 1.5 cm), most major organs begin their basic development.

Weeks 9–12: This is the transition from embryo to **fetus**. The placenta takes over hormone production, allowing the corpus luteum to regress. Facial features refine. The kidneys start producing urine, and spontaneous movements begin. External genitalia begin to show differentiation. At 12 weeks, the fetus is about 2.5 inches long, and the heartbeat is usually audible with a Doppler.

Development of Major Systems

Each organ system undergoes remarkable development in this trimester:

- **Cardiovascular system**: First to function; circulation begins early to sustain organ growth.

- **Nervous system**: Rapid neural tube closure is critical by week 6; brain vesicles begin to form.

- **Digestive & respiratory systems**: Basic tube formation, branching of bronchi, and liver/bile duct formation begin.

- **Musculoskeletal system**: Bones begin to ossify; limb buds develop into recognizable arms and legs.

- **Reproductive system**: Gonads form; external genitalia start differentiating by week 11–12.

➢ **Critical Risk Periods and Teratogenic Sensitivity**

- The first trimester is the **most vulnerable period** for teratogenic effects. Exposure to harmful substances — such as alcohol, certain medications (e.g., isotretinoin, thalidomide), and infections (e.g., rubella, cytomegalovirus) — can result in structural abnormalities.

- The role of **folic acid** in preventing neural tube defects underscores the importance of **preconceptional supplementation**, especially because neural tube closure happens before most women know they are pregnant.

➢ **Diagnostic and Clinical Milestones**

Modern obstetrics has equipped us with tools to track these invisible developments:

- **Ultrasound** at 6–7 weeks can confirm intrauterine pregnancy and cardiac activity.

- **Beta-hCG levels** help detect early viability or diagnose ectopic/molar pregnancies.

- **Nuchal Translucency (NT) scan**, combined with **biomarkers** (PAPP-A, free β-hCG), forms the cornerstone of first-trimester aneuploidy screening.

This window is also the ideal time for **genetic counseling**, **risk stratification**, and **planning prenatal follow-ups**.

➤ **Clinical Significance**

Many pregnancy complications originate in this trimester:

- Miscarriages
- Ectopic pregnancy
- Hyperemesis gravidarum
- Molar pregnancy
- Embryonic demise

Timely detection through scheduled checkups, ultrasounds, and bloodwork can mitigate long-term risks. Emotional reassurance during this time is just as crucial, especially for women with previous losses or high-risk factors.

*In summary, the first trimester is a **silent architect of life**. Everything from the **heart's rhythm to the brain's wiring** is initiated during these few weeks. By highlighting these milestones, we emphasize a new standard in pregnancy care — **proactive, precise, and deeply aware of the invisible** changes unfolding within.*

This chapter lays the groundwork for deeper understanding in upcoming sections — from prenatal diagnostics to maternal nutrition — always keeping in mind that the **inverted pyramid of antenatal care** begins at the very top: **the earliest weeks of life.**

(B) First Trimester Screening and Investigations — and Therefore the Importance of Early Booking

In the realm of obstetrics, the saying *"well begun is half done"* couldn't be more relevant than in the first trimester. This early phase is not only about confirming pregnancy — it's about establishing a **baseline** for everything that follows. The early weeks offer a fleeting but powerful window to screen for risks, prevent complications, and optimize outcomes. Unfortunately, many pregnancies remain unbooked until the second trimester, thereby missing the most **preventive and predictive** phase of antenatal care.

➤ Ideal Timing for First Antenatal Booking

The first antenatal visit should ideally occur **before 10 weeks** of gestation. Early booking is not just a formality — it's an entry point into the world of prenatal diagnostics and maternal-fetal medicine. This visit serves multiple purposes:

- Confirming pregnancy viability
- Estimating accurate gestational age
- Detecting risk factors
- Counseling for nutrition, lifestyle, and supplementation
- Planning a personalized follow-up schedule

At this stage, the fetus is small, but the decisions are big — and so is the impact.

➤ Baseline Investigations in Early Pregnancy

A comprehensive profile is created during the first visit to understand the mother's physiological status. Some of the most vital investigations include:

- **Complete Blood Count (CBC):** Detects anemia, infection, platelet count.
- **Blood Grouping and Rh Typing:** Prevents Rh incompatibility and isoimmunization.
- **Blood Sugar Testing:** Screens for overt diabetes.
- **Urine Routine and Culture:** Checks for asymptomatic infections, proteinuria.
- **LFT, RFT:** Checks for liver and renal functions.
- **Thyroid Profile (TSH):** Maternal hypothyroidism is linked to miscarriage and poor neurodevelopment.
- **HIV, HBsAg, VDRL, HCV:** Essential for early management, to prevent vertical transmission.
- **Rubella IgG:** Immunity status determines need for postpartum vaccination.
- **Toxoplasmosis/CMV/Herpes (TORCH):** Done selectively, based on history and local protocol.

➤ **Ultrasound Screening in the First Trimester**

Ultrasound is a cornerstone of early obstetric care. It allows us to:

- **Confirm intrauterine pregnancy**
- **Assess viability** (fetal pole, cardiac activity)
- **Determine gestational age** (crown-rump length is the most accurate method)
- **Detect multiple gestation**
- **Identify early complications** (blighted ovum, ectopic pregnancy, subchorionic hemorrhage)

Later in the first trimester (11–13.6 weeks), the **Nuchal Translucency (NT) scan** becomes a crucial part of prenatal screening.

First Trimester Combined Screening: NT Scan + Dual Marker

The combined first trimester screening involves:

- **Ultrasound NT measurement**
- **Serum markers:**
  - Pregnancy-associated plasma protein-A (PAPP-A)
  - Free β-hCG

This screen identifies risk for:

- **Down syndrome (Trisomy 21)**
- **Trisomy 18 (Edward's syndrome)**
- **Trisomy 13 (Patau syndrome)**

A high NT, especially when combined with altered markers, flags the need for further testing: **NIPT (non-invasive prenatal testing)** or **invasive testing** like CVS (chorionic villus sampling).

This risk-based approach reduces unnecessary anxiety, empowers informed choices, and allows time for advanced diagnostics — if needed.

Case Insight:

Let's consider Mrs. X, a 29-year-old woman who booked her pregnancy at 6 weeks because she had a prior miscarriage. Her early screening revealed severe hypothyroidism and Rh-negative status. She received immediate care — thyroid correction and Anti-D immunoglobulin at the right time. Today, she's a mother to a healthy baby girl. If she had booked later, the outcome might have been different.

***In summary**, the **first trimester is not just a gestational phase** — it's a critical phase of **decision-making, diagnostics, and disease prevention**. Early booking empowers obstetricians and families to make evidence-based decisions at a time when fetal development is most vulnerable yet most adaptable.*

"Screening is not about fear — it's about foresight."

(C) The Role of Nutrition and Supplementation — In General and in Relation to Organogenesis and Teratogenic Risk

The first trimester is a silent revolution in a woman's body. While externally subtle, internally, **organogenesis — the formation of organs — is in full swing**. This process, which largely occurs between **weeks 3 and 8**, is exquisitely sensitive to both nutritional support and toxic exposures. In this context, nutrition becomes not just a maternal concern but a **lifelong investment in the health and potential of the unborn child**.

> **Understanding Organogenesis: A Vulnerable Yet Powerful Phase**

Organogenesis begins shortly after implantation and continues through the embryonic stage, laying the blueprint for the heart, brain, spine, kidneys, limbs, and more. By the end of **week 8**, most major organs are formed and begin rudimentary functioning.

This is the **most sensitive time to nutritional deficits** or teratogenic exposure. A deficiency during this phase doesn't just delay development — it can cause irreversible structural defects. This is why **nutritional counseling and supplementation must begin preconceptionally or as early as possible** in pregnancy.

> **Key Nutrients in the First Trimester: What Builds a Healthy Baby**

Let's break down the essential nutrients and their roles in fetal development *(RDA includes dietary content + supplements):*

1. Folic Acid

- **Role**: Prevents neural tube defects (NTDs) like spina bifida and anencephaly.
- **Critical Window**: 3–6 weeks post-conception.
- **RDA**: 400–600 mcg/day (up to 4 mg for high-risk women).
- **Sources**: Green leafy vegetables, legumes, fortified grains.
- **Note**: Neural tube closes before most women realize they're pregnant, hence preconceptional folate is vital.

2. Iron

- **Role**: Formation of red blood cells, oxygen delivery, fetal brain development.
- **RDA**: 27 mg/day.
- **Sources**: Red meat, legumes, spinach, fortified cereals.
- **Deficiency Effects**: Intrauterine growth restriction (IUGR), preterm birth, maternal fatigue.

3. Iodine

- **Role**: Thyroid hormone synthesis, essential for neurodevelopment.
- **RDA**: 220 mcg/day.
- **Sources**: Iodized salt, dairy, seafood.
- **Deficiency Risks**: Cretinism, low IQ, miscarriage.

4. Vitamin D

- **Role**: Bone development, immune function.
- **RDA**: 600 IU/day (up to 2000 IU in deficiency).
- **Sources**: Sunlight, fortified dairy, egg yolks.

- **Deficiency Risks**: Skeletal deformities, maternal preeclampsia.

5. Calcium

- **Role**: Fetal bone and tooth development, maternal bone protection.
- **RDA**: 1000–1200 mg/day.
- **Sources**: Milk, yogurt, cheese, green vegetables.

6. Omega-3 Fatty Acids (DHA)

- **Role**: Brain and eye development.
- **Sources**: Fatty fish, flaxseed, chia seeds.
- **Recommendation**: 200–300 mg DHA/day in pregnancy supplements.

7. Protein and Calories

- **Protein RDA**: 1.1 g/kg/day.
- **Increased Caloric Needs**: +300 kcal/day by the end of the trimester.
- **Sources**: Lentils, meat, dairy, tofu.

➢ **Prenatal Supplements: What's in a Pill?**

Prenatal multivitamins help ensure no nutritional gaps exist, especially in women with nausea, food aversions, or limited access to fresh foods.

An ideal first-trimester prenatal supplement per day should include:

- Folic acid: 400–800 mcg
- Iron: 27 mg
- Iodine: 150 mcg
- Vitamin D: 600 IU
- Calcium: 1000–1200 mg

- DHA (if included): 200–300 mg

*(Guidelines by **WHO, ICMR, and FIGO** emphasize starting these supplements ideally before conception or as soon as pregnancy is confirmed. **Iron, calcium if not tolerated in first trimester due to nausea, should be started after 12- 14 weeks.**)*

➢ **When Nutrition Fails: Teratogenic Risks and Outcomes**

Certain nutritional deficiencies are directly linked to structural malformations or cognitive deficits:

Deficiency	Teratogenic Outcome
Folate	Neural tube defects (NTDs)
Iodine	Cretinism, developmental delay
Vitamin D	Skeletal deformities, rickets
Iron	IUGR, premature birth
Omega-3 (DHA)	Poor neurodevelopment

*Even excesses can be harmful. For example, **Vitamin A >10,000 IU/day** is associated with **craniofacial and heart defects** — making balanced intake vital.*

➢ **What to Avoid: Nutritional Teratogens and Harmful Foods**

During the first trimester, mothers must be cautious of food-borne illnesses and nutritional toxins. During first trimester pregnant women should generally **avoid raw or uncooked foods, unpasteurized dairy, excessive caffeine, and high mercury fish (e.g. shark, swordfish).** While some myths about papaya and carrot exist, they are not scientifically supported as teratogenic.

Specific Foods to Avoid:

1.Raw or Uncooked Foods: This includes raw or undercooked meat, poultry, fish and eggs. These can harbor bacteria like Listeria, Salmonella, and E. coli, which can cause serious infections and complications during pregnancy.

2.Unpasteurized Dairy Products: Soft cheeses, unpasteurized milk can also contain Listeria bacteria, which can be harmful.

3.High-Mercury Fish: Certain fish-like swordfish, shark and king mackerel contain high levels of mercury, which can be harmful to a developing fetus's nervous system (Neurotoxic).

4.Raw Sprouts: Raw or lightly cooked bean sprouts can also harbor bacteria like Listeria and Salmonella.

5.Unwashed Produce: Wash fruits and vegetables thoroughly to remove potential contaminants like pesticides which can harm and also parasites that can cause toxoplasmosis.

6.Excessive Caffeine: While moderate caffeine intake is generally considered safe, excessive consumption (>200 mg/day) has been linked to an increased link of miscarriage especially in early pregnancy and low birth weight later.

7.Alcohol: Alcohol consumption during pregnancy can cause serious developmental problems in the fetus. (Fetal Development Spectrum Disorder).

8.Unripe or Semi-Ripe Papaya: While ripe papaya is generally safe, unripe or semi-ripe varieties contain latex and papain, which can cause uterine contractions and potentially lead to miscarriage.

➢ **Contextual Considerations: Not One Diet Fits All**

Many factors influence maternal nutrition:

- **Vegetarian/Vegan diets**: May require B12, iron, DHA supplements.
- **Cultural beliefs**: Some women avoid certain foods in early pregnancy.
- **Low socioeconomic status**: Poor access to fresh or fortified foods.

Public health efforts should include **fortification programs, nutritional education**, and **targeted supplementation schemes** to bridge gaps.

➢ **A Small Change, A Big Impact**

*In summary, the first trimester represents **a narrow window** when nutrition can either protect or endanger the forming fetus. Unlike genetic risks, **nutrition is modifiable** — a unique chance to improve outcomes with relatively simple interventions.*

Every tablet of folic acid, every balanced meal, and every avoided toxin during these weeks creates the foundation of life itself. It's not just prenatal care — it's **preemptive medicine**, driven by knowledge, awareness, and love.

CHAPTER IV: EARLY RISK STRATIFICATION

"The more we know early in pregnancy,

the better we can plan and prevent complications.

Knowledge is the first step towards

a safer pregnancy."

-Anonymous

(A) Advanced Screening Protocols

Advanced screening protocols have revolutionized the way we approach antenatal care by allowing for the early detection and monitoring of potential complications. The goal of these protocols is not only to diagnose conditions but to predict and prevent adverse outcomes, thereby improving maternal and fetal health. In this section, we will explore the evolution and current state of advanced screening techniques, focusing on their role in enhancing early risk stratification.

Evolution of Screening Protocols

Historically, antenatal screening was limited to basic tests such as maternal serum screening for Down syndrome or ultrasound scans at specific stages of pregnancy. Over the years, advancements in medical technology have led to the development of more sophisticated protocols that can identify a wider range of potential risks much earlier in pregnancy. The increased availability of non-invasive, high-precision methods has allowed healthcare providers to screen for multiple conditions with greater accuracy.

Types of Advanced Screening Methods

There are several key types of advanced screening methods that have been incorporated into modern antenatal care protocols. These include:

1. First Trimester Maternal Serum Screening and Nuchal Translucency (NT) by Ultrasound: A Detailed Overview

In the first trimester of pregnancy, **maternal serum screening** combined with **nuchal translucency (NT) ultrasound** is a critical approach for early detection of certain chromosomal abnormalities, most notably **Down syndrome (trisomy 21)**, **trisomy 18**, and **trisomy 13**. Together, these tests form a vital part of the **first-trimester screening** process. This section provides an in-depth explanation of both screening tests, how they work together, and their significance in prenatal care.

First Trimester Maternal Serum Screening

Maternal serum screening involves a blood test performed during the first trimester (typically between **11 and 13.6 weeks** of gestation) to measure the levels of specific substances in the mother's blood. These substances include:

- **Pregnancy-Associated Plasma Protein A (PAPP-A):**
  PAPP-A is a protein produced by the placenta during pregnancy. Low levels of PAPP-A can be an indicator of an increased risk of **Down syndrome** and other chromosomal conditions, as well as adverse pregnancy outcomes like preeclampsia, growth restriction, and preterm birth.

- **Human Chorionic Gonadotropin (hCG):**
  hCG is a hormone produced by the placenta that helps maintain the pregnancy. Elevated levels of hCG are

often associated with **Down syndrome**, while lower-than-normal levels may indicate a risk for **trisomy 18** or **miscarriage**.

How the Maternal Serum Screening Works

- The blood test measures the levels of **PAPP-A** and **hCG** (and sometimes other substances, such as **free beta-hCG**) in the maternal bloodstream.

- The results are combined with other factors like the **mother's age**, **weight**, and **ethnicity**, to calculate the **risk** for certain genetic conditions.

- The results are typically expressed as risk ratio, and the ratio closer to 1 suggest a higher likelihood of the condition. For example, a ratio of 1: 250 or lower may indicate a high-risk result, requiring further investigations, while ratio of 1: 1000 or higher might suggest a low-risk result.

Key Points:

- **Advantages**: This test is simple, quick, and minimally invasive (just a blood draw). It helps identify women who may be at high risk for certain genetic disorders.

- **Limitations**: This is a **screening test**, not a diagnostic test. It identifies risk but cannot definitively diagnose a condition. False positives and false negatives can occur.

Nuchal Translucency (NT) Ultrasound

Nuchal translucency (NT) refers to the fluid-filled space at the back of a developing baby's neck, visible on ultrasound. The **NT scan** is typically performed between **11 and 13.6 weeks** of pregnancy and is used to measure the thickness of this area. An increased NT measurement can be a sign of potential genetic conditions, including **Down syndrome (trisomy 21)**, **trisomy 18**, **trisomy 13**, and other chromosomal or structural abnormalities.

How NT Ultrasound Works

- During an NT scan, the sonographer or expert sonologist uses high-resolution ultrasound to measure the **nuchal translucency**—the space behind the fetal neck.

- The size of this space is measured in **millimeters**, and abnormal thickening of the NT may indicate the need for further diagnostic evaluation.

- Along with the NT measurement, the **nasal bone** is also assessed, as its absence or underdevelopment can further increase the risk for chromosomal conditions.

The **cutoff level for Nuchal Translucency (NT)**

It is generally determined based on the measurement of the **nuchal translucency** in millimeters (mm) at **11 to 13.6 weeks** of gestation. The NT measurement reflects the fluid-filled space at the back of the fetal neck, and increased thickness can be a marker for **chromosomal abnormalities** like **Down syndrome (trisomy 21)**, **trisomy 18**, and **trisomy 13**, as well as other structural anomalies.

Typical Cutoff Levels for NT Measurement

- **Normal NT Range:**
  - For **Down syndrome** and other chromosomal abnormalities, a **normal NT measurement** is typically less than **2.5 mm**. This is considered a **low-risk** result for chromosomal abnormalities.

- o An NT measurement of **2.5 mm or less** is often interpreted as within the **normal range** and typically does not indicate an increased risk of these conditions.

- **Increased NT Measurement**:
  - o An NT measurement of **greater than 2.5 mm** is considered **increased** and may indicate an **increased risk** for **chromosomal abnormalities**, particularly **Down syndrome** and **trisomy 18**.
  - o An NT measurement greater than **3.0 mm** is often considered **high-risk** and warrants further diagnostic testing (e.g., **NIPT**, **amniocentesis**, or **CVS**) to confirm the presence of any chromosomal abnormalities or structural defects.

- **Risk Interpretation Based on NT Measurement**
  - o **NT ≤ 2.5 mm**: Generally considered within the **normal range**, with a lower likelihood of major chromosomal abnormalities.
  - o **NT > 2.5 mm but ≤ 3.0 mm**: May indicate an **increased risk** for chromosomal abnormalities, but still within a range where further screening tests (e.g., **NIPT** or **combined serum screening**) are recommended to refine risk assessment.
  - o **NT > 3.0 mm**: Strongly suggests a **higher risk** for **Down syndrome**, **trisomy 18**, **trisomy 13**, or other abnormalities, and **diagnostic testing** (e.g., **CVS** or **amniocentesis**) is typically recommended.

- **Important Considerations:**
  - o **Gestational Age**: NT measurement should be taken at the correct gestational age (between **11 and 13.6 weeks**), as NT values can vary with the development of the fetus.
  - o **Maternal Factors**: The interpretation of NT measurements also depends on factors like **maternal age, ethnicity**, and **history of previous pregnancies** with chromosomal abnormalities. These factors are

integrated with NT data for a more comprehensive risk assessment.

- o **Other Ultrasound Markers**: NT measurements are often combined with other ultrasound markers, such as **nasal bone presence** and **fetal heart function**, and combined with serum markers like **PAPP-A** and **free β-hCG** in a comprehensive risk model.

- **Key Takeaways**
  - o **NT ≤ 2.5 mm** is typically **normal**, and higher measurements (greater than 3.0 mm) are considered **high-risk**.
  - o **Limitations**: NT ultrasound alone cannot definitively diagnose a chromosomal abnormality, but it can indicate an increased risk NT measurement should **always be considered in conjunction with other diagnostic tools, such as serum markers and maternal factors,** to assess the overall risk of chromosomal abnormalities. In cases where NT measurements are abnormal, further diagnostic tests such as **non-invasive prenatal testing (NIPT), amniocentesis,** or **chorionic villus sampling (CVS)** may be recommended.
  - o **Advantages**: NT ultrasound is a non-invasive method and provides immediate results. It also helps assess the baby's overall development, including the presence or absence of the nasal bone.

*In practice, the cutoff values may slightly vary based on the **sonologist's expertise**, the **quality of the ultrasound equipment**, and the **specific guidelines** followed by different medical institutions, but the general ranges described above are widely used in clinical settings.*

Combined First-Trimester Screening: Maternal Serum + NT Ultrasound

When the **maternal serum screening** is combined with the **nuchal translucency ultrasound**, it provides a more comprehensive risk assessment. This combined approach has a **higher sensitivity and accuracy** in detecting chromosomal abnormalities than each test used separately.

How the Combined Test Works

- **Step 1: Maternal Serum Screening** (Blood Test):
  - The blood sample is taken from the mother between **11 and 13.6 weeks** of pregnancy.
  - Levels of **PAPP-A** and **hCG** are measured, and these values are combined with the mother's age and other factors to assess risk.

- **Step 2: Nuchal Translucency Ultrasound**:
  - The NT measurement is taken during an ultrasound performed between **11 and 13.6 weeks** of pregnancy.
  - The **nuchal translucency measurement** is combined with the blood test results, age, and other factors to calculate a risk ratio for chromosomal abnormalities.

- **Step 3: Risk Calculation**:
  - The results of the blood test and the NT ultrasound are input into a **mathematical model** that generates a **risk score** for the fetus having conditions like Down syndrome, trisomy 18, or trisomy 13.
  - This combined test offers improved sensitivity (ability to detect true positives) and reduces the likelihood of false positives compared to either test alone.

Risk Calculation Formula

The formula for risk calculation considers the following factors:

- **Maternal age**
- **PAPP-A and hCG levels**
- **Nuchal translucency measurement**
- **Gestational age**

- **Ethnicity**
- **Weight and other personal factors**

For example, a woman who is **35 years old**, with an **increased NT measurement** and **low PAPP-A levels**, will have a higher risk of a chromosomal abnormality than a woman of the same age with normal NT and PAPP-A levels.

Key Points:

Advantages: The combined approach has **higher accuracy** in detecting conditions like Down syndrome (Trisomy 21) and **trisomy 18** in the first trimester. It also offers a less invasive method of risk assessment, as opposed to amniocentesis or CVS, which carry a risk of miscarriage.

Limitations: While the combined screening test provides a highly accurate risk assessment, it is still a **screening** rather than a diagnostic test. A positive result only indicates an **increased risk** and does not confirm a condition. False positives and false negatives are still possible.

Sensitivity and Specificity

- **Sensitivity** refers to the ability of the test to correctly identify those with the condition (true positives). A higher sensitivity means that the test is good at detecting the condition in those who actually have it.

- **Specificity** refers to the ability of the test to correctly identify those without the condition (true negatives). A higher specificity means that the test is good at ruling out those who do not have the condition.

First Trimester Screening (Maternal Serum + NT) for Down Syndrome (Trisomy 21)

For **Down syndrome** (trisomy 21), the sensitivity and specificity of the combined first-trimester maternal serum screening with NT ultrasound are as follows:

- **Sensitivity**: The combined test for Down syndrome has a **sensitivity of around 85-90%**. This means that the test can correctly identify 85-90% of pregnancies affected by Down syndrome.

- **Specificity**: The specificity of the combined screening for Down syndrome is typically **90-95%**. This means that the test can correctly identify 90-95% of pregnancies that do not have Down syndrome, minimizing the number of false positives.

First Trimester Screening for Trisomy 18

For **trisomy 18**, which is a severe chromosomal condition, the combined maternal serum and NT screening has the following performance characteristics:

- **Sensitivity**: The sensitivity for trisomy 18 is generally **85-90%**, similar to Down syndrome, although it can vary depending on factors like maternal age and the quality of the ultrasound.

- **Specificity**: The specificity for trisomy 18 is generally **95% or higher**, which indicates that the combined test is very good at correctly identifying pregnancies that are not affected by trisomy 18.

First Trimester Screening for Trisomy 13

For **trisomy 13**, a condition that results in severe developmental issues and is often fatal within the first year, the sensitivity and specificity are as follows:

- **Sensitivity**: The combined screening has a **sensitivity of about 70-80%** for trisomy 13. This is slightly lower than for trisomy 21 and 18, but it is still a useful screening tool for detecting this rare condition.

- **Specificity**: The specificity for trisomy 13 is generally **90-95%**, making the test relatively effective at ruling out this condition in unaffected pregnancies.

Key Points

- **Overall Sensitivity**: When combined, the first-trimester maternal serum screening and NT ultrasound are highly sensitive for **detecting Down syndrome (85-90%)** and **trisomy 18 (85-90%)**, while being somewhat less sensitive for **trisomy 13 (70-80%)**.

- **Overall Specificity**: The specificity is high, typically **90-95%**, which helps minimize false positives and ensures that women with low-risk results are less likely to undergo unnecessary follow-up testing.

Advantages of the Combined Screening

- **Increased Sensitivity**: The combination of the **serum markers** (PAPP-A, hCG) and **NT ultrasound** improves sensitivity compared to using either test alone. This allows for a higher detection rate of chromosomal abnormalities.

- **Reduction of False Positives**: With high specificity, this combined screening reduces the likelihood of **false positive results**, thereby minimizing the number of women who would need invasive diagnostic procedures (such as amniocentesis or CVS) following an abnormal screening result.

- **Early Risk Assessment**: By performing this test early in pregnancy (around **11-13.6 weeks**), healthcare providers can assess the risk of certain conditions early on and offer appropriate counseling and follow-up care.

Limitations

- **False Positive Rate**: Despite the high specificity, there is still a **false positive rate** of around 5-10%, meaning some women with no abnormalities will receive a positive result and may undergo unnecessary testing.

- **Not Diagnostic**: This is a **screening test**, not a diagnostic test. A positive result suggests an increased risk but does not confirm a condition. Diagnostic tests such as **NIPT**, **amniocentesis**, or **CVS** may be needed to confirm the diagnosis.

Conclusion

*The first-trimester **maternal serum screening** combined with **nuchal translucency ultrasound** provides a powerful tool **for early detection of chromosomal abnormalities** and other fetal conditions. This combined approach improves the sensitivity and accuracy of screening, offering a comprehensive risk assessment at a time when early intervention can make a significant difference. However, it is essential for healthcare providers to communicate clearly with expectant parents about the purpose and limitations of these tests, emphasizing that they **are designed to assess risk, not provide definitive diagnoses.** In cases of high-risk results, **additional diagnostic tests** can offer more conclusive answers and guide subsequent decision-making.*

2. Ultrasound Imaging:

Advances in ultrasound technology have enabled clearer, high-resolution imaging, allowing for better evaluation of fetal anatomy and development at earlier stages of pregnancy. First-trimester ultrasounds are now used to **assess fetal growth**, **detect structural abnormalities**, and **measure nuchal translucency**, which is an important marker for chromosomal conditions.

Advantages: Ultrasound is a non-invasive, widely accessible tool that provides valuable information about fetal anatomy and can also detect early signs of complications like ectopic pregnancy, multiple pregnancies, and uterine abnormalities.

Limitations: While ultrasound is invaluable in diagnosing fetal structural abnormalities, it may not always be able to detect all genetic disorders or subclinical conditions, which is where other screening methods play a complementary role.

In the first trimester, with the use of high-resolution ultrasound machines and the expertise of an experienced sonologist, a **variety of structural anomalies can** be detected. **Early detection** is critical as it allows for early intervention and management, which can **significantly improve outcomes for both the mother and the fetus**. Below are the key structural anomalies that can be detected during the first trimester using advanced ultrasound technology:

Neural Tube Defects (NTDs)

- **Anencephaly**: This is a condition where the brain and skull do not develop properly. It is usually evident during the first trimester ultrasound through the absence of the skull and brain structures.
- **Spina Bifida**: A condition in which the spine does not close properly, leading to potential nerve damage. In the first trimester, a sonologist may detect spinal abnormalities or signs of a defect in the closure of the neural tube.

Cardiac Abnormalities

- **Congenital Heart Defects (CHDs)**: The basic structure of the heart and major blood vessels can be assessed using first-trimester ultrasound. The sonologist may detect:
- **Septal defects** (e.g., atrial or ventricular septal defects)
- **Hypoplastic left heart syndrome** (underdeveloped left side of the heart)
- **Transposition of the great arteries** (where the two main arteries of the heart are swapped)

While detailed **heart structures are best visualized** in the second trimester **(20 – 22 weeks),** basic abnormalities in heart development, such as irregularities in the heart rate, flow, and positioning, can be identified early on.

Cleft Lip and Palate

- **Cleft Lip**: A condition where there is an opening or gap in the upper lip, often extending into the nose. A skilled sonologist can detect this anomaly as early as 12 weeks gestation.
- **Cleft Palate**: A condition where the roof of the mouth does not close completely. While cleft palate may be more difficult to detect in the first trimester, advanced ultrasound techniques can reveal signs of abnormal oral cavity development.

Abnormalities in Limb Development

- **Limb Reduction Defects**: These include conditions where one or more limbs are underdeveloped or absent. Early ultrasound can detect limb abnormalities, such as missing or shortened limbs (e.g., amelia or hemimelia), as well as polydactyly (extra fingers or toes).
- **Clubfoot**: A condition where the foot is twisted out of its normal position. This can often be identified through first-

trimester ultrasound, especially when combined with other signs of abnormal limb positioning.

Abnormalities of the Abdomen

- **Gastroschisis**: A defect in the abdominal wall where the intestines are found outside the fetus's body. This anomaly can be detected early with high-resolution ultrasound.
- **Omphalocele**: A condition where abdominal organs protrude into the base of the umbilical cord. It is usually identifiable in the first trimester and can be detected through careful assessment of the abdominal contents.
- **Bladder Extrophy**: A rare condition where the bladder develops outside the body. It may be identified on an early ultrasound as an abnormal appearance of the fetal abdomen.

Renal Anomalies

- **Renal Agenesis (Absence of Kidneys)**: In cases of unilateral or bilateral renal agenesis, the kidneys may not develop properly or may be absent. This can be detected as early as the first trimester with high-resolution ultrasound.
- **Multicystic Dysplastic Kidney (MCDK)**: This condition involves the presence of cysts in one or both kidneys, which can lead to kidney dysfunction. It can often be observed on early ultrasound as abnormal kidney structures.

Abnormalities of the Gastrointestinal System

- **Duodenal Atresia**: A blockage of the duodenum (part of the small intestine), which can be detected on ultrasound by observing fluid-filled loops of the intestine or a "double bubble" sign.
- **Hirschsprung's Disease**: A condition where the large intestine lacks nerve cells, resulting in bowel obstruction.

Although the diagnosis is often made later in pregnancy, signs of abnormal bowel movement or distension can sometimes be observed early.

Structural Abnormalities of the Spine

- **Scoliosis**: An abnormal curvature of the spine can sometimes be detected early if the ultrasound shows a misalignment of the vertebrae.
- **Spinal Dysraphism**: This refers to a condition where the spine does not form properly. While some forms of dysraphism, such as spina bifida, are detected in the first trimester, more complex spinal malformations may become clearer later in pregnancy.

Placental Abnormalities

- **Placenta Previa**: This occurs when the placenta is located low in the uterus and covers the cervix, which can lead to complications during labor. Although it's more **commonly diagnosed later**, in some cases, it may be seen early on.
- **Placental Abnormalities**: Abnormalities like placental accreta (where the placenta grows too deeply into the uterine wall) can be suspected if certain ultrasound findings suggest unusual attachment patterns.

Structural Abnormalities in the Face and Skull

- **Microcephaly**: This condition, characterized by an abnormally small head, can sometimes be detected early through ultrasound measurements of the fetal head.
- **Hydrocephalus**: Excess fluid in the brain can be suspected if there is abnormal enlargement of the ventricles. This may be detected early if the sonologist notices an abnormally large head size or other signs of fluid buildup.

Fetal Growth Retardation (FGR)

- **Growth Retardation**: In cases where the fetus is not growing at the expected rate, an expert sonologist can identify growth restrictions early in pregnancy. This can sometimes be identified through measurements of the fetal crown-rump length, head circumference, or abdominal circumference.

Structural Abnormalities in the Neck

- **Cystic Hygroma**: This is a fluid-filled sac that can develop in the neck region due to lymphatic system malformations. It can be detected on a first-trimester ultrasound as an abnormal fluid collection.

Twins or Multiple Gestation

- **Monochorionic and Dichorionic Twins**: Early ultrasound can distinguish between types of twin pregnancies, with implications for management, as monochorionic twins are at higher risk for complications like twin-to-twin transfusion syndrome (TTTS).

Conclusion

*While the first trimester is generally focused on the early detection of major structural anomalies, it's important to note that **some abnormalities may not be detectable until later in pregnancy (18 – 20 weeks anomaly scan).** However, with the combination of **high-resolution ultrasound technology and the expertise of an experienced sonologist**, a wide range of structural anomalies can be identified early, allowing for timely interventions, planning, and counseling for the expecting parents. **Early detection is crucial in managing these conditions,** improving maternal and fetal outcomes, and offering informed choices for the next steps in the pregnancy.*

3. Non-Invasive Prenatal Testing (NIPT)

Non-Invasive Prenatal Testing (NIPT) is one of the most significant advancements in prenatal screening. It has revolutionized early detection by providing a non-invasive, highly accurate, and safe method to assess the risk of certain chromosomal abnormalities in the fetus, including Down syndrome (trisomy 21), trisomy 18, trisomy 13, and sex chromosome abnormalities. NIPT analyzes fetal DNA found in the maternal blood, providing an early, risk-free alternative to traditional invasive diagnostic procedures like amniocentesis or chorionic villus sampling (CVS), which carry a small risk of miscarriage.

How NIPT Works

NIPT works by analyzing **cell-free fetal DNA (cfDNA)** that circulates in the maternal bloodstream. During pregnancy, small fragments of the fetus's DNA naturally enter the mother's bloodstream, coming from the placenta. These fetal DNA fragments are detectable as early as the 10th week of pregnancy. By sequencing these fragments, NIPT can identify chromosomal abnormalities without the need for invasive procedures.

- **Blood Collection**: A simple blood sample is drawn from the mother, typically from the arm. The blood contains both maternal DNA and fetal DNA fragments.
- **DNA Extraction and Sequencing**: The fetal DNA is isolated from the maternal blood sample, and advanced sequencing techniques, such as massively parallel sequencing or microarray analysis, are used to examine the genetic material.
- **Risk Assessment**: The amount of fetal DNA from specific chromosomes is compared to reference levels. Any anomalies, such as extra or missing chromosomes, can be detected based on deviations from the expected proportions.

- **Results**: The results are typically available within 7-10 days. The test provides a risk assessment (e.g., high or low risk) for specific genetic conditions based on the analysis of the fetal DNA.

Conditions Detected by NIPT

NIPT can be used to screen for a variety of genetic conditions. The most commonly screened conditions include:

- **Down Syndrome (Trisomy 21)**:
  Down syndrome is a genetic condition caused by an extra copy of chromosome 21. It is the most commonly tested condition with NIPT, with detection rates exceeding 99%.

- **Trisomy 18**:
  Trisomy 18 (Edwards syndrome) is a genetic disorder caused by an extra chromosome 18. It leads to severe developmental delays, and most affected infants die within the first year of life. NIPT has high sensitivity for this condition.

- **Trisomy 13**:
  Trisomy 13 (Patau syndrome) is caused by an extra chromosome 13 and results in severe intellectual and physical disabilities. NIPT can identify this condition with a high degree of accuracy.

- **Sex Chromosome Abnormalities**:
  NIPT can also detect abnormalities related to sex chromosomes, such as **Turner syndrome (monosomy X), Klinefelter syndrome (XXY)**, and other variations in the number of X and Y chromosomes.

- **Microdeletion Syndromes**:
  Some NIPT tests offer screening for rare **microdeletion syndromes**, such as **22q11.2 deletion**

syndrome (DiGeorge syndrome). However, these screenings are less common and have lower detection rates compared to trisomy testing.

- **Other Aneuploidies**:
  Some NIPT panels also screen for additional conditions caused by the presence of extra or missing chromosomes, such as **triploidy** (three sets of chromosomes instead of two).

Advantages of NIPT

- **Non-Invasive**:
  Unlike amniocentesis or CVS, NIPT carries no risk of miscarriage because it only involves a simple blood draw from the mother.

- **High Accuracy**:
  NIPT is highly accurate, with detection rates for trisomy 21 (Down syndrome) surpassing 99%, and detection rates for other trisomies like 18 and 13 generally around 97-98%. False-positive and false-negative results are rare.

- **Early Detection**:
  NIPT can be performed as early as the 10th week of pregnancy, providing earlier information about fetal health compared to traditional screening methods, which typically occur between the 11th and 14th weeks of pregnancy.

- **Reduced Need for Invasive Testing**:
  By providing highly accurate results, NIPT significantly reduces the need for invasive tests like amniocentesis and CVS, which can carry risks to both the mother and fetus.

- **Comprehensive**:
  NIPT can screen for multiple genetic conditions in one test, including both trisomies and sex chromosome abnormalities.

Limitations of NIPT

- **Not Diagnostic**:
  While NIPT is highly accurate in screening for genetic conditions, it is not diagnostic. A positive result indicates a high risk of a condition, but it does not confirm that the fetus has the condition. In cases of high-risk results, further diagnostic testing such as amniocentesis or CVS is recommended for confirmation.

- **Limited to Chromosomal Conditions**:
  NIPT primarily screens for chromosomal abnormalities. It does not assess other aspects of fetal health, such as structural defects (e.g., heart defects), neural tube defects, or other genetic disorders that may not be related to chromosomal issues.

- **False Positives/Negatives**:
  Although rare, false-positive and false-negative results can occur. A false-positive result means that the test suggests a chromosomal abnormality when there is none, while a false-negative result means that the test misses a condition that is actually present.

- **Limited Availability**:
  NIPT may not be available in all healthcare settings, particularly in low-resource areas. The test can also be costly, and not all insurance companies cover it, though this is changing as the test becomes more mainstream.

- **Ethical and Psychological Considerations**:
  NIPT provides highly sensitive information early in pregnancy, which can present ethical and psychological challenges. Parents must carefully consider how they want to proceed with the information they receive, particularly in cases of positive results.

Clinical Use and Guidelines

NIPT is typically recommended for women who are at higher risk of chromosomal abnormalities. This includes women who:

- Are 35 years or older, as maternal age being a known risk factor for genetic conditions.

- Have a history of previous pregnancies with chromosomal abnormalities.

- Have abnormal results from other prenatal screenings (e.g., serum screening or ultrasound).

- Are carrying twins or multiple fetuses (though NIPT's effectiveness is somewhat reduced in these cases).

- However, NIPT is becoming more widely available, and many guidelines now support its use for all pregnant women as a first-line screening tool due to its high accuracy and non-invasive nature.

Future Directions in NIPT

The future of NIPT is promising, with ongoing research aimed at expanding its scope. Researchers are exploring how NIPT can be used to detect additional conditions, such as:

- **Single-gene disorders** (e.g., cystic fibrosis, sickle cell anemia), though these are much more complex to detect and are not currently part of routine NIPT panels.

- **Fetal epigenetic changes** that could indicate an increased risk of conditions like autism or schizophrenia.

- As genetic testing technology continues to advance, it's expected that the scope of NIPT will continue to expand, offering more comprehensive prenatal screening options in the near future.

Conclusion

*Non-Invasive Prenatal Testing **(NIPT)** has undoubtedly transformed the landscape of prenatal care, providing pregnant women with an accurate, safe, and **early means of detecting chromosomal abnormalities.** With its high accuracy, non-invasive nature, and ability to detect multiple conditions, NIPT represents a major advancement in personalized maternal-fetal medicine. However, as with any screening test, it's essential for healthcare providers and expectant parents to **understand the limitations** and implications of the results and make informed decisions based on them.*

(B) The Latest Predictive Markers for Preeclampsia, GDM, and Aneuploidies

"In the journey of pregnancy,

early screening is not just a test;

it's the foundation of informed decisions

and healthier futures."

-Anonymous

Introduction

Predictive markers in pregnancy are increasingly being utilized to assess the risk of various complications early in the gestation period. These markers help healthcare providers identify pregnancies at high risk for **preeclampsia**, **gestational diabetes mellitus (GDM)**, and **aneuploidies** (chromosomal abnormalities), enabling timely interventions that can significantly improve maternal and fetal outcomes. In this section, we will discuss the latest predictive markers for each of these conditions, focusing on their clinical applications and how they improve early risk stratification.

1. Predictive Markers for Preeclampsia

Preeclampsia is a hypertensive disorder of pregnancy that affects 5-8% of pregnancies globally. It can result in serious complications for both the mother and fetus, such as **preterm birth**, **fetal growth restriction**, and **maternal organ damage**. Early identification of high-risk pregnancies allows for closer monitoring and preventive measures.

Latest Predictive Markers for Preeclampsia

Several biomarkers and clinical markers are now being used to predict the risk of developing preeclampsia:

- **Placental Growth Factor (PlGF)**:
  o **PlGF** is a protein produced by the placenta that plays a crucial role in the growth of blood vessels. **Low levels of PlGF** are associated with an increased risk of preeclampsia, **particularly in the second trimester.** It has become one of the most significant biomarkers in predicting preeclampsia. (Normal: > 100 pg/mL).

  o **Clinical Application**: Measurement of **PlGF** levels in the maternal blood, typically done after 20 weeks, is useful for identifying women at high risk for **early-onset preeclampsia** (before 34 weeks gestation). A **low PlGF level** indicates poor placental perfusion and may prompt closer monitoring or early intervention.

- **Soluble Fms-Like Tyrosine Kinase-1 (sFlt-1)**:
  o **sFlt-1** is an anti-angiogenic factor that inhibits the action of vascular endothelial growth factor (VEGF), which is necessary for proper blood vessel formation. Elevated levels of sFlt-1 have been linked to preeclampsia, as it disrupts the balance of angiogenesis (blood vessel formation) and leads to endothelial dysfunction.

  o **Clinical Application**: **sFlt-1** is often used in combination with **PlGF** for early detection. A **high sFlt-1/PlGF ratio** is predictive of **early-onset preeclampsia** and helps determine the likelihood of developing the condition within weeks.

Interpretation of sFlt-1/PlGF Ratio

- **High sFlt-1/PlGF Ratio (≥85)**: This indicates an **increased likelihood** of **early-onset preeclampsia,** especially in women who have additional risk factors for the condition. These women may require more frequent monitoring and possible early interventions (e.g., the use of low-dose aspirin, blood pressure monitoring, and close surveillance of fetal growth).

- **Normal or Low sFlt-1/PIGF Ratio (<38)**: A ratio below this value suggests a **lower risk** of developing preeclampsia. However, it is not a definitive guarantee, and ongoing monitoring is still important for women with other risk factors or clinical signs that might suggest preeclampsia.

- **Intermediate sFlt-1/PIGF Ratio (38-85)**: An intermediate ratio is considered **indeterminate**, and the results should be interpreted in conjunction with other clinical factors and tests. These patients may require follow-up testing and monitoring to assess their risk over time.

Clinical Utility of sFlt-1/PIGF Ratio

- **Early Prediction of Preeclampsia**:
  The sFlt-1/PIGF ratio is particularly useful for **early prediction** of **preterm preeclampsia** (before 34 weeks), which has a higher risk of maternal and fetal complications, **the test is typically performed between 24 to 28 weeks of gestation.**

- **Timely Intervention**:
  By identifying high-risk pregnancies earlier, healthcare providers can initiate preventive measures such as **low-dose aspirin** (which has been shown to reduce the risk of preeclampsia in high-risk women) and provide close monitoring for signs of preeclampsia (e.g., blood pressure monitoring, fetal growth scans, etc.).

- **Supplementing Traditional Risk Factors**:
The sFlt-1/PIGF ratio adds value to traditional clinical risk factors like **maternal age**, **history of preeclampsia**, and **preexisting conditions (e.g., hypertension)**. It helps refine risk assessment and personalize care for pregnant women.

- **Better Outcomes**:
Early identification of preeclampsia can lead to better management and outcomes by allowing healthcare providers to make timely decisions regarding **delivery timing, fetal monitoring**, and **maternal treatment**.

Conclusion

*The **sFlt-1/PIGF ratio** is a useful tool in predicting **preeclampsia**, particularly **early-onset preeclampsia**, by identifying women at high risk earlier in pregnancy. The **cutoff of ≥85** is typically used to identify high-risk women who need closer monitoring and intervention. A **ratio** <38 generally suggests a **low-risk** pregnancy for preeclampsia. This test, in combination with other clinical factors and screening tools, can improve early detection and management, ultimately helping to reduce the risks associated with preeclampsia for both mother and baby.*

- **Angiogenic Factors**:
  - **Angiogenic proteins** like **VEGF (vascular endothelial growth factor)** and **endoglin** also play roles in predicting preeclampsia. Imbalances in these factors can indicate vascular abnormalities.

  - **Clinical Application**: Measurement of **endoglin** levels, especially in combination with PIGF, helps identify high-risk pregnancies earlier than traditional methods.

- **Uterine Artery Doppler Ultrasound**:
  - o **Uterine artery Doppler** in the first trimester (usually between (11 – 14 weeks) is an important and non-invasive screening used to assess the risk of preeclampsia (PE) and fetal growth restriction (FGR). It evaluates uteroplacental blood flow and can help identify woman at higher risk for adverse pregnancy outcomes.

  - o **Rationale**
    Preeclampsia is a placental disorder characterized by defective trophoblastic invasion of maternal spiral arteries, leading to high-resistance uteroplacental circulation. A doppler study in early pregnancy can detect the abnormal vascular resistance.

  - o **Procedure**
    - Performed using transabdominal or transvaginal ultrasound with color and pulsed doppler.
    - The uterine artery is visualized at the level of internal os where it crosses the external iliac artery.
    - Pulsatile index (PI) is the key measurement, reflecting resistance to blood flow.
    - Both left and right uterine arteries are assessed, and the mean PI is calculated.
    - Presence and absence of an early diastolic notch is also noted (a persistent notch after the first trimester is abnormal.)

  - o **Interpretation**
    - High mean arterial PI (> 95th percentile) and/or presence of bilateral notching suggest increased risk.
    - The lower the PI, the better the placentation.
    - These findings are especially significant when combine with:
      - ✓ Maternal risk factors (e.g., chronic hypertension, previous PE.)

     ✓ Biochemical markers (PAPP-A, PIGF)
     ✓ Mean arterial pressure (MAP).

- **Clinical Utility**
  - Part of the first trimester combined screening for preeclampsia and FGR.
  - Helps stratify women into low and high-risk groups.

- **Limitations**
  - Screening tool only – not diagnostic.
  - Operator-dependent and requires standardization of technique.
  - Predictive value is higher for early-onset PE than late-onset.

- **Conclusion**

  *First trimester uterine artery Doppler is a valuable component of multimodal screening for preeclampsia. **When combined with clinical and biochemical markers,** it allows **early identification and management of at-risk pregnancies**, particularly through low-dose aspirin prophylaxis.*

2. Predictive Markers for Gestational Diabetes Mellitus (GDM)

Gestational Diabetes Mellitus (GDM) is another common pregnancy complication, affecting around **2-10% of pregnancies**. GDM increases the risk of **preterm labor, macrosomia (large baby),** and **neonatal hypoglycemia**, among other complications. Identifying women at risk early allows for timely intervention and lifestyle changes to reduce the impact.

Available Predictive Markers for GDM

- **First-Trimester Glycated Hemoglobin (HbA1c)**:
  - o **HbA1c** reflects the average blood glucose levels over the past 2-3 months. Elevated levels **(≥5.7%)** in early pregnancy can predict the development of GDM later in the pregnancy.
  - o **Clinical Application**: Testing **HbA1c** in the **first trimester** can help identify women at risk for GDM, particularly those with a history of **obesity**, **family history of diabetes**, or **advanced maternal age**.

- **Fasting Plasma Glucose (FPG)**:
  - o **FPG** is a simple blood test that measures glucose levels after an overnight fast. Elevated levels of **fasting glucose** in early pregnancy (≥92 mg/dL) can be an indicator of future GDM.
  - o **Clinical Application**: An **FPG** test can help identify women with impaired glucose metabolism early in pregnancy, allowing for interventions like dietary counseling, exercise programs, or early glucose monitoring.

- **OGTT**
  OGTT is the **gold standard** for diagnosing gestational diabetes mellitus. It plays a pivotal role in identifying glucose tolerance during pregnancy, which can have significant maternal and fetal implications if left unmanaged.

Why OGTT for GDM??
GDM is a condition characterized by glucose intolerance first recognized during pregnancy. The placental hormones (like human placental lactogen, progesterone, cortisol, etc.) create a state of insulin resistance, especially in the second and third trimesters. Some women cannot compensate with increased insulin secretion, leading to hyperglycemia.

The OGTT helps identify this by evaluating how the body handles an oral glucose load, making it a functional assessment of glucose metabolism during pregnancy.

WHO/IADPSG Recommended OGTT Protocol (75g OGTT)
Conducted between 24 – 28 weeks of gestation (or earlier if risk factors are present.).

Procedure after overnight fasting:
- Fasting blood glucose
- 75g oral glucose load
- Blood glucose at 1 hour
- Blood glucose at 2 hours

Diagnostic threshold (based on IADPSG/WHO criteria):

- Fasting > 92 mg/dl (5.1 mmol/L)
- 1 hour > 180 mg/dl (10.0 mmol/L)
- 2 hour > 153 mg/dl (8.5 mmol/L)

Diagnosis of GDM is made if any one value is met or exceeded.

Why it Works??

- OGTT measures pancreatic beta-cell reserve and insulin resistance.
- Pregnancy is a metabolic stress test – OGTT reveals subclinical glucose intolerance not evident in fasting or postprandial glucose alone.

OGTT vs Other Screening Tests

- **Test:** OGTT
- **Advantage:** Gold standard, diagnostic
- **Limitations:** Time-consuming, patient preparation needed.

- o **Test:** Random blood glucose
- o **Advantage:** Easy, quick
- o **Limitations:** Low sensitivity

- o **Test:** Fasting Blood Glucose
- o **Advantage:** Good predictor of insulin resistance
- o **Limitations:** Misses postprandial hyperglycemia

- o **Test:** HbA1c
- o **Advantage:** Useful in pregestational diabetes
- o **Limitations:** Not sensitive enough for GDM

Variations in OGTT Approach

- o **DIPSI (India)** recommends a non-fasting 75g OGTT with a single 2-hour value > 140 mg/dl
- o Advantage: Practical in low resource settings
- o Criticized for **low sensitivity** compared to OGTT.

Clinical Significance of OGTT

Timely diagnosis via OGTT allows for interventions – diet, exercise, insulin therapy – to prevent complications such as:

- o Macrosomia
- o Preeclampsia
- o Shoulder dystocia
- o Neonatal hypoglycemia
- o Future risk of type 2 diabetes in mother and child

Indications for First Trimester Screening for GDM

Although the **OGTT** is usually performed in the second trimester, there are situations in which **early screening** for **GDM** might be appropriate:

High-Risk Women:
The **first trimester** is typically used for screening in women

who have a **higher risk** of developing **gestational diabetes**. This may include women who:

- o **Obesity (BMI ≥30 kg/m²)**: Obese women are at a higher risk of insulin resistance and may develop GDM earlier.

- o **History of GDM in a previous pregnancy**: Women who had GDM in a previous pregnancy are at an increased risk of developing it again in subsequent pregnancies.

- o **Family history of diabetes** (first-degree relatives with **type 2 diabetes**): A family history of diabetes increases the likelihood of insulin resistance during pregnancy.

- o **Advanced maternal age** (≥35 years): Older mothers are at a higher risk of developing GDM.

- o **Polycystic Ovary Syndrome (PCOS)**: Women with PCOS are at higher risk for insulin resistance and GDM.

- o **Previous large baby (macrosomia)**: Women who have had a previous baby weighing more than **9 lbs (4.1 kg)** may be at higher risk for developing GDM.

- o **Ethnicity**: Certain ethnic groups, such as **Hispanic**, **African American**, **Asian**, and **Native American** women, are at higher risk for GDM.

- **Homeostasis Model Assessment of Insulin Resistance (HOMA-IR)**:
  The **HOMA-IR** (Homeostatic Model Assessment of Insulin Resistance) is an indirect marker of insulin resistance, and it has emerged as a useful predictive tool for GDM – especially in early pregnancy or even preconceptionally in those with obesity or polycystic

ovarian syndrome (PCOS). High insulin resistance early in pregnancy has been associated with the development of GDM.

How it is Calculated??

HOMA-IR is calculated using fasting glucose and fasting insulin levels:

$$HOMA\text{-}IR = \frac{\text{Fasting Insulin x Fasting Glucose}}{405}$$

Why it is relevant to GDM

Pregnancy naturally induces insulin resistance, but in some women, pre-existing subclinical insulin resistance makes them more vulnerable to GDM. HOMA-IR, when measured early in pregnancy or preconceptionally, can help identify these high-risk women before overt hyperglycemia develops.

Clinical Significance

o Early Risk Stratifications: Women with elevated HOMA-IR (usually > 2.5) are more likely to develop GDM.

o Supplement to OGTT: HOMA-IR is not a replacement to OGTT but can guide early surveillance and personalized care.

o Clinical Application: Measurement of **HOMA-IR** can help identify women at increased risk for GDM, especially in those with obesity or polycystic ovary syndrome (PCOS).

Strengths and Limitations

> **Strengths:**
> - Simple, inexpensive
> - Useful in early pregnancy
> - Helps in risk prediction
>
> **Limitations:**
> - Not standardized across labs
> - Requires fasting sample
> - No universal cut-off for GDM

- **Serum Markers (C-Peptide, Insulin):**
  - Elevated **C-peptide** or **insulin** levels in early pregnancy can indicate insulin resistance, which is a precursor to GDM.

  - **Clinical Application**: Testing for **C-peptide** or **insulin** levels, along with fasting glucose, can help identify women at high risk for GDM before the traditional screening at 24-28 weeks.

3. Predictive Markers for Aneuploidies (Chromosomal Abnormalities)

Aneuploidies, such as **Down syndrome (trisomy 21)**, **trisomy 18**, and **trisomy 13**, are common chromosomal conditions associated with developmental delays, congenital anomalies, and early mortality. Detecting these conditions early in pregnancy allows for better management and decision-making.

Latest Predictive Markers for Aneuploidies

- **Non-Invasive Prenatal Testing (NIPT):**
  - **NIPT** is a groundbreaking test that analyzes cell-free fetal DNA circulating in the maternal blood. It can

screen for **trisomy 21, trisomy 18, trisomy 13**, and sex chromosome abnormalities with high accuracy.

- o **Clinical Application**: **NIPT** is considered the gold standard for detecting aneuploidies due to its **high sensitivity (99%)** and **specificity (99%)**, especially when used in combination with **maternal serum screening** and **NT ultrasound**. It is a non-invasive alternative to amniocentesis and CVS.

- **First-Trimester Serum Markers (PAPP-A and Free Beta-hCG)**:
  - o In addition to NIPT, **PAPP-A** (Pregnancy-Associated Plasma Protein A) and **free beta-hCG** are routinely measured in the first trimester to screen for aneuploidies. Low levels of PAPP-A and high levels of free beta-hCG are indicative of an increased risk of **Down syndrome** and **trisomy 18**.

  - o **Clinical Application**: These markers are part of the **first-trimester combined screening** with NT ultrasound and provide a valuable risk estimate for aneuploidies, especially when combined with maternal age and other factors.

- **Ultrasound Markers (Nuchal Translucency and Nasal Bone Presence)**:
  - o **Nuchal Translucency (NT)** is the fluid-filled space at the back of the fetus's neck, which can be measured by ultrasound. An **increased NT measurement** is associated with an increased risk for chromosomal abnormalities like **Down syndrome** and **trisomy 18**.

  - o **Nasal Bone Absence**: The absence or underdevelopment of the nasal bone during an NT ultrasound is an additional marker for an increased risk of **Down syndrome**.

- o **Clinical Application**: NT measurement, in combination with **serum markers** and **maternal age**, forms part of the first-trimester screening for **aneuploidies**, enhancing the accuracy of risk assessment.

- **Combined First-Trimester Screening**:
  - o The combination of **serum markers (PAPP-A, hCG), NT ultrasound**, and **maternal age** is used to assess the risk of aneuploidies in the first trimester. This screening is highly sensitive and provides a **risk ratio** for conditions like **Down syndrome**, **trisomy 18**, and **trisomy 13**.

  - o **Clinical Application**: This screening approach is widely used and provides an effective, non-invasive means of identifying high-risk pregnancies for chromosomal conditions early in the pregnancy.

Conclusion

*The latest predictive markers for **preeclampsia**, **gestational diabetes mellitus (GDM)**, and **aneuploidies** offer valuable insights into the risk assessment and early detection of these common pregnancy complications. By utilizing these markers, healthcare providers can identify pregnancies at high risk for adverse outcomes and implement appropriate interventions to improve maternal and fetal health. The continued advancement in biomarkers, along with the integration of new technologies like **NIPT**, is making it possible to detect and manage pregnancy complications more effectively than ever before.*

(C) How to Design Personalized Care Pathways for Better Pregnancy Outcomes

"The future of maternal care lies

in personalized pathways that prioritize

early intervention and precise monitoring."

-Anonymous

Introduction

When high-risk conditions such as **preeclampsia**, **GDM**, or **chromosomal abnormalities** are identified in the **first trimester**, it is crucial to design a **personalized care pathway** for the pregnant individual. These pathways involve more than just medical interventions; they also include lifestyle modifications, continuous monitoring, and regular counseling. The goal is to **optimize the health of both the mother and the fetus** by addressing the risk early on, allowing for preventive measures and timely interventions to be implemented.

1. Personalized Care Pathway for Preeclampsia

Preeclampsia is a pregnancy-related hypertensive disorder that can lead to serious maternal and fetal complications, including **eclampsia**, **organ failure**, and **preterm birth**. When high-risk factors for preeclampsia (e.g., elevated **sFlt-1/PIGF ratio**, abnormal **uterine artery Doppler**, or a family history) are identified in the first trimester, personalized care pathways can significantly improve the pregnancy outcome.

Steps in Designing a Care Pathway for High-Risk Preeclampsia:

- **Early Monitoring and Blood Pressure Control**:
  - **Frequent blood pressure monitoring** is essential in high-risk pregnancies. Ideally, blood pressure should be measured at **every visit**.

  - **Home blood pressure monitoring** may be encouraged, with instructions on how to track readings.

  - If **hypertension** is identified early, **antihypertensive medications** (e.g., **labetalol, nifedipine**) may be prescribed to keep blood pressure under control.

- **Aspirin Therapy**:
  - For women at high risk, especially those with previous **preterm preeclampsia, low-dose aspirin** (81 mg daily) should be initiated between **12 to 16 weeks** of pregnancy. Aspirin has been shown to reduce the risk of developing **preterm preeclampsia** and **fetal growth restriction**.

  - This should continue until **37 weeks** or the delivery of the baby.

- **Nutritional and Lifestyle Modifications**:
  - **Low-sodium diet** and **balanced nutrition** (rich in antioxidants, calcium, and magnesium) should be encouraged. Studies have shown that a **balanced diet** helps reduce the risk of **hypertension** in pregnancy.

  - **Weight management**: For overweight or obese women, a **moderate weight loss** plan before pregnancy (if possible) and healthy weight gain during pregnancy are essential.

- o **Physical activity**: Encouraging moderate physical activity, such as walking or prenatal yoga, can improve circulation and reduce stress.

- **Monitoring Fetal Growth**:
  - o **Regular fetal growth scans** (every 4-6 weeks) to monitor for signs of **fetal growth restriction (FGR)**, which is a common complication of preeclampsia.

  - o **Doppler ultrasound** for assessing placental blood flow may be performed to identify placental insufficiency.

- **Referral to Specialist Care**:
  - o Referral to an **obstetrician specializing in high-risk pregnancies** may be warranted for closer monitoring and additional interventions.

  - o If necessary, **hospital admission** may be required for **severe preeclampsia** management, including possible **early delivery**.

2. Personalized Care Pathway for Gestational Diabetes Mellitus (GDM)

Gestational diabetes mellitus (GDM) is another common condition that requires personalized care to prevent complications such as **macrosomia, preterm labor, neonatal hypoglycemia**, and **increased cesarean delivery rates**. Early identification of GDM risk allows for lifestyle modifications and glycemic control measures that can significantly improve maternal and fetal health.

Steps in Designing a Care Pathway for High-Risk GDM:

- **Early Screening and Monitoring**:
  - If **early screening** for GDM (such as **HbA1c**, **FPG**, or **75g OGTT**) identifies a high risk, **more frequent glucose monitoring** should be implemented.
  - **Self-monitoring of blood glucose** (SMBG) at home, with instructions on how to test and when, is critical for effective management.
  - **Continuous glucose monitoring (CGM)** may be an option for some high-risk women.

- **Dietary Modifications**:
  - **Carbohydrate counting** and **meal planning**: Work with a **dietitian** to help the mother make appropriate dietary changes that include **low-glycemic index foods**, **high-fiber**, and **protein-rich foods**.
  - Encourage **small, frequent meals** to help maintain steady blood glucose levels throughout the day.
  - Educate about the impact of different food choices on blood sugar, focusing on limiting simple sugars and refined carbohydrates.

- **Physical Activity**:
  - Encourage **moderate exercise** such as walking or swimming, which can help improve insulin sensitivity.
  - Regular **physical activity** can also help with weight management and reduce the likelihood of **macrosomia**.

- **Medication**:
  - If **diet and exercise** do not effectively control blood glucose, **insulin therapy** may be needed.
  - Alternatively, medications like **metformin** or **glyburide** may be considered if **insulin** is not desirable or feasible.

- o **Close monitoring** of blood glucose levels is essential to adjust insulin doses or oral medications as required.

- **Monitoring for Other Pregnancy Complications**:
  - o **Frequent fetal growth scans** are important to assess for **macrosomia** and monitor fetal development.
  - o **Delivery planning**: Women with GDM are at an increased risk for **shoulder dystocia** during delivery due to fetal macrosomia, so careful delivery planning is necessary.

- **Postpartum Follow-Up**:
  Women with **GDM** should be **screened for type 2 diabetes** postpartum, typically at **6 weeks** after delivery, since they are at increased risk for developing type 2 diabetes later in life.

3. Personalized Care Pathway for Aneuploidies (Chromosomal Abnormalities)

If high risk for **aneuploidies** (e.g., **Down syndrome**, **trisomy 18**, **trisomy 13**) is identified early, personalized care pathways involve counseling, further diagnostic testing, and planning for possible outcomes.

Steps in Designing a Care Pathway for High-Risk Aneuploidies:

- **Follow-Up Diagnostic Testing**:
  - o If **NIPT** or **combined first-trimester screening** identifies high risk for **aneuploidies**, confirmatory diagnostic tests like **amniocentesis** or **chorionic villus sampling (CVS)** may be offered. These tests provide definitive information about whether the fetus has a chromosomal abnormality.

- o **Genetic counseling** should be offered to the parents to discuss the risks, benefits, and implications of further testing, as well as potential outcomes.

- **Decision-Making and Counseling**:
  - o After receiving results from diagnostic testing, **genetic counseling** becomes essential to help the parents make informed decisions about their pregnancy.
  - o **Emotional and psychological support** should be offered, as a diagnosis of a chromosomal abnormality can be overwhelming.

- **Monitoring and Early Interventions**:
  - o If the pregnancy continues with an **aneuploidy diagnosis**, specialized **neonatal care** planning is needed.
  - o For conditions like **Down syndrome**, early intervention services (e.g., **speech therapy**, **physical therapy**, **occupational therapy**) can be initiated once the baby is born to improve developmental outcomes.

- **Supportive Care and Options**:
  - o If the condition is serious, such as **trisomy 18** or **trisomy 13**, where there may be a very limited life expectancy, **palliative care** and **end-of-life planning** may be discussed with the family, depending on the condition and their wishes.

Conclusion

*When high risks for **preeclampsia, GDM,** or **aneuploidies** are detected in the first trimester, **personalized care pathways** are essential for improving pregnancy outcomes. These pathways focus on early detection, continuous monitoring, preventive interventions (such as **aspirin therapy** or **insulin management**), and ongoing counseling and support. By customizing the approach based on the individual's risk profile and medical history, healthcare providers can ensure better management and outcomes for both the mother and the baby.*

CHAPTER V: SAFE MEDICATIONS AND SUPPLEMENTS

"The first gift we give our children is not love,

but life — and life begins with

the silent strength of nutrients

that shape their tomorrow."

-Anonymous

(A) First Checkpoint: Securing the Medication Landscape

Introduction

Pregnancy introduces profound physiological changes in a woman's body, altering drug absorption, metabolism, and excretion.

Thus, **reviewing all current medications** at the **earliest prenatal visit or preconception consultation** is critical. This process helps identify medications that may:

- Pose teratogenic risks

- Need dosage adjustments

- Require discontinuation or substitution

Goal: To ensure both maternal health and fetal safety by rationalizing drug therapy.

Why Medication Review is Important in Pregnancy

- **Teratogenicity Risk**: Some drugs can cause congenital malformations, especially if continued during organogenesis (first trimester).

- **Pharmacokinetic Changes**: Pregnancy alters drug absorption, plasma volume, hepatic metabolism, and renal clearance.

- **Maternal Disease Management**: Some conditions (e.g., epilepsy, hypertension, diabetes) require continued management, but with safer alternatives.

- **Avoid Polypharmacy**: Minimize unnecessary medications to lower cumulative risk.

- **Detect Self-Medication Risks**: Over-the-counter drugs, herbal products, and traditional remedies might not be safe.

Step-by-Step Approach to Reviving Current Medications

- **Detailed Medication History**
  - **Prescription drugs**: Chronic illness medications (e.g., for hypertension, diabetes, epilepsy, psychiatric disorders).

  - **Over-the-counter (OTC) drugs**: Painkillers, cold medicines, antacids, etc.

  - **Supplements**: Multivitamins, herbal remedies, Ayurvedic medicines.

  - **Substance use**: Alcohol, nicotine, recreational drugs.

Identify Potentially Harmful Drugs

- Cross-check against known **teratogenic drug lists** (e.g., FDA Pregnancy Risk Categories, updated guidelines).

- Special attention to:
    - **ACE inhibitors**
    - **Isotretinoin**
    - **Warfarin**
    - **Valproate**
    - **Tetracyclines**
    - **Methotrexate**

Risk-Benefit Analysis

- **Continue**: If the benefit to the mother clearly outweighs the potential risk to the fetus (e.g., insulin in diabetes).

- **Switch**: Safer alternatives (e.g., replace ACE inhibitors with labetalol for hypertension).

- **Discontinue**: If the medication is non-essential or harmful (e.g., isotretinoin for acne).

Counseling the Patient

- Explain why medication changes are necessary.

- Reinforce **not stopping essential medications abruptly** (e.g., stopping antiepileptics without planning can be dangerous).

- Discuss risks of untreated maternal conditions versus drug risks.

Special Considerations

- **First Trimester**: Highest sensitivity period (**organogenesis),** critical to avoid harmful drugs.

- **Chronic Illnesses**:
  Asthma, diabetes, hypertension, psychiatric disorders require individualized planning.

- **Antibiotic Use**: Ensure antibiotics prescribed are safe (e.g., avoid **tetracyclines**, prefer penicillin class if needed).

Conclusion

*Reviving current medications is not merely about stopping drugs; it is a **careful balance between maintaining maternal health and ensuring fetal safety**. A proactive, systematic review during **early pregnancy** or ideally **preconception** can significantly reduce adverse pregnancy outcomes and improve maternal confidence and compliance.*

Sample Case Study: Medical Review in Early Pregnancy

Mrs. A, a 28-year-old woman, presented for her first antenatal visit at 7 weeks of pregnancy. She had a history of **epilepsy**, diagnosed at the age of 18, and was currently taking **sodium valproate (500 mg twice daily)** for seizure control.

- **Detailed Medication History**
  o Prescription drugs: Sodium valproate
  o No other medications or supplements
  o No smoking or alcohol history

- **Identify Risk**
  - Sodium valproate is a **high-risk teratogen**, associated with:
    - ✓ Neural tube defects (e.g., spina bifida)
    - ✓ Facial dysmorphisms
    - ✓ Cognitive developmental delays

- **Risk-Benefit Analysis**
  - Continuing valproate risks serious congenital malformations.
  - Abrupt withdrawal increases seizure risk, endangering both mother and fetus.

- **Management Plan**
  - **Immediate referral to a neurologist** specializing in pregnancy care.
  - Gradual tapering of valproate under close supervision.
  - **Switch to lamotrigine**, a safer alternative with lower teratogenic risk.
  - **High-dose folic acid supplementation (5 mg daily)** initiated to reduce neural tube defect risk.

- **Counseling**
  - Mrs. A was counseled on the risks of her current medication and the need for close seizure monitoring.
  - She was reassured about the availability of safer alternatives and regular follow-up was arranged.

- **Key Learning Points from this Case:**
  - Some chronic conditions **must** be managed throughout pregnancy, but **drug choice matters**.
  - **Early booking** and **medication review** can prevent serious birth defects.
  - **Specialist collaboration** (e.g., obstetrician + neurologist) is critical in high-risk medication adjustments.

o   **Patient education and involvement** improve compliance and outcomes.

Summary Box: Reviving Current Medications

- ***Early Review is Critical****: Always review all prescription, over-the-counter, and herbal medications at the **first prenatal visit** or **preconception consultation***.

- ***Identify and Assess Risks****: Flag any drugs known to have **teratogenic potential**, and evaluate the **risk-benefit** ratio for continuing them.*

- ***Make Safe Adjustments****: Where possible, **discontinue**, **switch to safer alternatives**, or **adjust doses** under specialist guidance.*

- ***Counsel and Involve the Patient****: Explain risks, benefits, and safe options clearly. Empower the mother to actively participate in her treatment decisions.*

- ***Collaborate and Monitor****: Coordinate care with relevant specialists (e.g., neurologists, cardiologists) and ensure **ongoing monitoring** of maternal and fetal health.*

(B) Category-Wise Drug Safety in Pregnancy

"Always verify with updated clinical guidelines.

Always prioritize maternal-fetal safety

over symptom management."

-Anonymous

Introduction

Not all drugs are equally harmful during pregnancy — but understanding which ones are **safe, risky, or absolutely contraindicated** is critical for both doctors and mothers. This subchapter will organize drug safety in pregnancy **category-wise**, giving readers a **clear, actionable framework**.

Evolution of Drug Safety Classification

Earlier, the **FDA Pregnancy Risk Categories (A, B, C, D, X)** were widely used, but they have now been **replaced** by the **Pregnancy and Lactation Labeling Rule (PLLR)** to give more detailed risk information.

For simplicity and understanding, we will first explain the **traditional ABCDX system** (still familiar globally) and then highlight **modern recommendations**.

1. Understanding Traditional FDA Categories

- **Category A (Safest):** *Controlled studies show no risk to fetus.*
  - **Folic Acid**: Prevents neural tube defects.
  - **Levothyroxine**: For hypothyroidism, critical to continue.

- **Category B (Generally Safe):** *No evidence of risk in humans; animal studies may show risk*
  - o **Penicillin antibiotics**: e.g., Amoxicillin.
  - o **Metformin**: In gestational diabetes management.
  - o **Ondansetron**: For nausea and vomiting (use under guidance).

- **Category C (Use with Caution***): Risk cannot be ruled out; use only if benefits justify risks.*
  - o **Gabapentin**: For neuropathic pain.
  - o **Fluoxetine**: An SSRI for depression.
  - o **Salbutamol**: For asthma (benefit usually outweighs risk).

- **Category D (Positive Risk, Use Only If Needed):** *Positive evidence of human fetal risk; may still be used in life-threatening situations.*
  - o **Phenytoin**: For epilepsy control.
  - o **ACE Inhibitors**: Severe risks if used in second/third trimester (renal dysgenesis).
  - o **Tetracyclines**: Cause tooth discoloration and skeletal abnormalities.

- **Category X (Contraindicated):** *Contraindicated in pregnancy; risk clearly outweighs benefit.*
  - o **Isotretinoin: Severe birth defects.**
  - o **Warfarin**: Risk of fetal bleeding and malformations.
  - o **Methotrexate**: Abortifacient and teratogenic.
  - o **Thalidomide:** Cause **phocomelia**, which include shortened or missed limbs, malformed limbs, and other abnormalities such as internal organ damage, including heart, kidney and gastrointestinal issues. **Thalidomide tragedy led to the removal of the drug from the market in many countries.** (*Thalidomide was introduced in 1953 as sedative and medication for morning sickness* **without having being tested on pregnant women.**)

2. Newer Approach: Pregnancy and Lactation Labeling Rule (PLLR)

- Instead of simple A-X categories, **PLLR** requires detailed sections:
  - Pregnancy (including labor and delivery)
  - Lactation
  - Females and Males of Reproductive Potential

- Gives more **nuanced information**: real-world clinical data, animal study results, risk management advice
  - **For Example**:
    Instead of just "Category C," a drug label now explains:
    "Animal studies show fetal risk; human data insufficient; recommend use only if benefit outweighs risk."

3. Practical Use in Clinical Decision-Making

- **Category A and B** drugs are generally preferred.
- **Category C** drugs require cautious benefit-risk analysis.
- **Category D and X** drugs should be **avoided or replaced** unless absolutely necessary (D) or completely contraindicated (X).
- **Individualize treatment**: no one-size-fits-all.

Special Caution with Herbal and OTC Products
Many natural products are **unregulated** and **not safe** despite marketing claims. e.g., high-dose Vitamin A supplements (risk of craniofacial defects).

In summary, drug safety is a spectrum, not an absolute black-and-white decision in pregnancy. By knowing category-wise safety, healthcare providers can make informed, individualized decisions ensuring both maternal health and fetal safety.

(C) Foundations of a Healthy Beginning: Essential Supplements for the First Trimester

"Supplements are not mere prescriptions;

they are acts of nurturing and protecting

future generations".

-Anonymous

Introduction

The first trimester is the **most critical phase** for fetal development — organogenesis, neural tube formation, placental establishment, and initial metabolic programming all happen during these first 12 weeks. Even minor deficiencies in this period can have **lifelong impacts** on fetal health.

Hence, certain **essential supplements** are universally recommended to **optimize maternal and fetal outcomes**.

Key Essential Supplements

1. Folic Acid — *The Guardian Against Neural Tube Defects*

- **Dosage**:
  - *Low-risk pregnancy*: 400–600 micrograms daily.
  - *High-risk pregnancy* (history of NTDs, epilepsy, obesity, diabetes): 4–5 mg daily.
- **Start**:
  Ideally **preconception one month before planning for pregnancy**, but at least as soon as pregnancy is confirmed.
- **Duration**:
  Continue through the **first trimester**, and often throughout pregnancy.

- **Benefits**:
  - o Reduces the chances of neural tube defects such as spina bifida, anencephaly by 70%.
  - o Reduces risk of congenital heart defects.

2. Iron — *Building Blocks for Blood*

- **Dosage**:
  30–60 mg elemental iron daily (WHO recommendation).
- **Start**:
  In the **first trimester** if anemic; otherwise often **started after 12–14 weeks to avoid worsening nausea.**
- **Benefits**:
  - o Prevents maternal anemia.
  - o Supports expanding blood volume and fetal iron stores.

3. Calcium — *Bones, Muscles, Heart Development*

- **Dosage**:
  1000–1200 mg daily (from diet + supplements).
- **Start**:
  Typically started later (after first trimester), but if maternal intake is low, early supplementation can be considered.
- **Benefits**:
  - o Prevents maternal bone demineralization.
  - o Lowers risk of preeclampsia.

4. Vitamin D — *Essential for Immunity and Bone health*

- **Dosage**:
  600–800 IU daily (higher if deficiency proven).
- **Start**:
  Early pregnancy, continued throughout.
- **Benefits**:

o   Supports calcium absorption.
o   Improves maternal and neonatal bone health.

5. Iodine — *Brain Development Booster*

- **Dosage**:
  150–250 micrograms daily.
- **Start**:
  Early pregnancy or preconception.
- **Benefits**:
  o   Crucial for fetal brain and nervous system development.
  o   Prevents cretinism and intellectual disabilities.

6. Omega-3 Fatty Acids (DHA) — *Brain and Eye Development*

- **Dosage**:
  200–300 mg DHA daily.
- **Start**:
  First trimester or even earlier if planning pregnancy.
- **Benefits**:
  o   Supports cognitive and visual development.
  o   May reduce risk of preterm birth.

7. Multivitamin-Mineral Supplements — *When Needed*

- In women with poor dietary intake, vomiting, or high-risk pregnancies.
- Should **not exceed** upper safe limits of fat-soluble vitamins (D, E, K).

- ➤ **Special Situations Needing Individualized Supplementation:**
  - **High-dose folic acid**: Epilepsy, previous child with NTD, obesity.
  - **Additional vitamin B12**: Vegetarians/vegans.

- **Higher Vitamin D**: Obese women or those with limited sun exposure.
- **Zinc, Magnesium**: Specific cases based on deficiency.

Key Practice Points:

- **Start early** — Preconception or as soon as pregnancy is confirmed.

- **Compliance counseling** — Many women stop supplements due to nausea; alternate dosing times or gentle formulations can help.

- **Avoid mega doses** — More is not always better; excesses can be harmful.

- **Prefer prescribed and evidence-based supplements** — Avoid over-the-counter self-medication.

Conclusion

*Supplements are not a luxury during pregnancy — they are **essential foundations** for **healthy fetal programming** and **maternal well-being**. The first trimester offers a **critical window** to correct and optimize nutrient supply when it matters most.*

CHAPTER VI: NAVIGATING NUTRITION PITFALLS AND RISKY HABITS IN EARLY PREGNANCY

The early stages of pregnancy are often surrounded by a whirlwind of advice, traditions, and personal experiences. While many recommendations are rooted in genuine care, not all align with modern medical understanding. Making the right nutritional and lifestyle choices in the first trimester is crucial — not only to ensure the healthy development of the baby but also to safeguard the well-being of the mother.

In this chapter, we will explore three key areas where confusion often arises:

- Common myths about dietary restrictions,
- The hidden dangers of alcohol, tobacco, and environmental exposures,
- The influence of cultural and religious beliefs on food and lifestyle choices.

By dispelling myths, highlighting real risks, and respecting cultural sensitivities, we aim to empower mothers-to-be with clarity, confidence, and practical guidance for this delicate and vital phase of life.

(A) Busting Dietary Myths of the First Trimester

The first trimester often brings a flood of well-meaning advice from family, friends, and even social media. However, not all dietary guidance stands up to scientific scrutiny. Let's separate myths from reality to help expectant mothers make informed, confident decisions about their nutrition. While the intention behind these practices was likely protective, not all of them hold up under modern scrutiny.

1. Myth: "Eating papaya and pineapple causes miscarriage."

✓ **Reality:**
Unripe papaya contains **latex,** which may **cause uterine contractions, if consumed in large quantities**, but **ripe papaya** in moderation is **generally safe**. In fact, ripe papaya is rich in vitamins like A, C, and folate, and is safe in moderate amounts. The **caution** lies only with **unripe papaya,** which could **potentially be risky** due to the presence of **latex enzymes**.
Similarly, **pine apple** contains **bromelain,** which in very high, **concentrated doses could soften the cervix,** but normal dietary intake is unlikely to reach such levels. **No direct link to miscarriage has been proven in practical dietary contexts.**
Scientific evidence does not support blanket bans unless allergies or specific medical conditions exist.

2. Myth: Carrot unsafe during first trimester

✓ **Reality:**
Yes, carrots **are safe** during pregnancy, including the first trimester, because they contain **beta-carotene**, a provitamin A compound. The key difference is:

- **Preformed vitamin A (Retinol)** – found in **animal-based food (e.g. liver, fish oils, dairy), fortified foods and supplements – can be teratogenic in high doses.**

- **Beta Carotene (precursor of vitamin A)** – found in **plant-based foods (e.g. carrot, sweet potatoes, spinach) – is not teratogenic,** it has to get converted to retinol first to be biologically active. The body regulates its conversion to active vitamin A based on the need. One cannot overdose on vitamin A from beta carotene through dietary food – the body converts only as much as it needs, especially in deficiency states.

3. Myth: "Pregnant women should eat for two."

✓ **Reality:**
While nutritional needs do increase, energy requirements rise only modestly in the first trimester. Overeating can lead to unhealthy weight gain and increase the risk of gestational diabetes and hypertension.

4. Myth: "Spicy food can harm the baby."

✓ **Reality:**
Spicy foods may cause heartburn or nausea in mothers, but do not directly harm the developing fetus. Moderation and individual tolerance are key, as nausea and heartburns are already prevalent in first trimester.

5. Myth: "Avoid all seafood."

✓ **Reality:**
Low-mercury seafood like **salmon, shrimp, and tilapia** provide essential **omega-3 fatty acids** beneficial for fetal **brain development.** Only **high-mercury fish like shark, swordfish, and king mackerel should be strictly avoided.**

6. Myth: "Pregnant women must completely avoid caffeine."

✓ **Reality:**
Moderate caffeine intake (**up to 200 mg/day** — about one 12-oz cup of coffee) is considered **safe** according to major health organizations like **ACOG** and **WHO.**

Final 5 Key Takeaways:

- Traditional wisdom should not be dismissed, but it should be filtered through scientific understanding.

- Moderation and food safety are more important than absolute bans.
- Individual allergies, medical history, and tolerance levels should guide food choices.

- Eating a varied, balanced diet supports optimal fetal development.

- Always consult a healthcare provider before making significant dietary change.

(B) Silent Threats: Alcohol, Tobacco/Smoking, and Environmental Hazards

"Simple lifestyle adjustments and awareness

can drastically minimize environmental

risks to the unborn child."

-Anonymous

While dietary choices are often the focus of early pregnancy advice, there are other, often overlooked, threats that can silently impact fetal development. Substances like alcohol and tobacco, along with certain environmental exposures, may seem harmless in small amounts but can have profound and lasting effects on pregnancy outcomes. In this section, we will explore these hidden dangers and understand why complete awareness and precaution are essential from the very beginning.

Alcohol: No Safe Limit

- **Impact on the Fetus:**
  - Alcohol easily crosses the placenta and can interfere with the normal growth and development of the baby.

  - Risks include Fetal Alcohol Spectrum Disorders (FASD) — causing brain damage, facial deformities, growth problems, and lifelong cognitive disabilities.

- **Current Scientific Standpoint:**
  - No amount of alcohol is considered safe at any stage of pregnancy **(CDC, ACOG, WHO guidelines).**

o Even occasional or "social drinking" can pose a risk, especially during the critical early stages of organ formation.

- **Key Takeaway:**
Complete avoidance of alcohol is the safest choice during pregnancy.

Tobacco and Smoking: Poison in Every Puff

- **Impact on Pregnancy:**
  o Smoking restricts oxygen supply to the baby by damaging blood vessels and reducing placental function.

  o Increases the risk of miscarriage, ectopic pregnancy, preterm birth, low birth weight, and stillbirth.

- **Secondhand Smoke:**
  o Even passive exposure to cigarette smoke significantly raises risks of poor fetal growth and sudden infant death syndrome (SIDS).

- **Key Takeaway:**
Pregnant women should avoid both active smoking and secondhand smoke exposure entirely.

Environmental Hazards: Hidden Dangers Around Us

- **Common Environmental Exposures:**
  o Pesticides and insecticides

  o Heavy metals like lead and mercury

  o Household cleaning chemicals (ammonia, bleach fumes)

- o Air pollution and industrial chemicals (BPA, phthalates)

- **Potential Effects:**
  - o Birth defects, developmental delays, immune dysfunction, low birth weight, and risk of miscarriage.

- **Precautionary Measures:**
  - o Use natural, pregnancy-safe cleaning products.

  - o Wash fruits and vegetables thoroughly to reduce pesticide exposure.

  - o Limit exposure to polluted environments and toxic substances.

  - o Prefer well-ventilated spaces and filtered drinking water.

*In Summary, alcohol, tobacco, and environmental toxins can have **permanent, avoidable** impacts on pregnancy outcomes. Early precaution, **complete avoidance of harmful substances**, and conscious environmental choices are vital **for a healthy pregnancy.***

(C) Cultural Beliefs and Religious Practices: Respecting Traditions While Safeguarding Health

"Traditions connect us to our roots,

while science lights the path

to a safer future"

Pregnancy is not just a biological journey — it is deeply woven into the cultural and spiritual fabric of societies around the world. Traditional food practices, fasting rituals, and spiritual customs often reflect generations of accumulated wisdom, love, and care for expectant mothers. However, while many of these customs are nurturing, some may unintentionally conflict with modern medical knowledge.

In this section, we will explore how cultural and religious practices can be honored thoughtfully, while ensuring that maternal and fetal health always remains the highest priority.

1. Traditional Food Beliefs: Nurturing or Risky?

- **Positive Traditions:**
  - Special postpartum foods (like laddoos, herbal decoctions, and ghee-based preparations) often have nourishing intentions.

  - Culturally recommended foods like lentils, dairy, and nuts provide excellent nutrition when consumed appropriately.

- **Potential Risks:**
  - Certain foods are culturally labeled as **"hot"** or **"cold"** and may be unnecessarily restricted during pregnancy (e.g., bananas, curd, citrus fruits).

o Blind avoidance without medical reasoning can deprive mothers of essential nutrients like folic acid, calcium, and vitamin C.

- **Balanced Guidance:**
  o Respect traditional beliefs, but cross-check critical dietary restrictions with healthcare advice.

  o Encourage inclusion of scientifically proven beneficial foods in culturally acceptable forms.

2. Religious Fasting During Pregnancy: Devotion vs. Health Needs

- **Common Practices:**
  o Fasting during religious observances (e.g., **Navratri, Ramadan**) is common in many cultures.

- **Medical Concerns:**
  o Prolonged fasting can cause dehydration, low blood sugar, nutrient deficiencies, and stress for both the mother and fetus.

  o Risk is higher during the first trimester when fetal organ development is underway.

- **Modern Medical Advice:**
  o Ideally, fasting should be avoided or modified during pregnancy under medical supervision.

  o If a woman strongly wishes to fast, modified fasting plans (e.g., frequent small nutritious meals, maintaining hydration) should be discussed with the doctor.

3. Bridging Tradition and Modern Science: A Respectful Approach

- **Cultural Sensitivity:**
  o Encourage conversations between healthcare providers, pregnant women, and family elders with a spirit of mutual respect.

  o Understand the emotional, spiritual, and social importance of traditional practices.

- **Scientific Empowerment:**
  o Provide clear, empathetic education about why certain adjustments are needed during pregnancy.

  o Promote *"safe traditions"* — adapting customs in a way that retains spiritual meaning but protects maternal and fetal health.

- **Empowering Mothers:**
  o Equip pregnant women with both medical knowledge and the confidence to make informed choices without disrespecting cultural roots.

In Summary, traditions and religious practices offer emotional strength but should be balanced with scientific health needs. **Respecting culture while safeguarding health is not a compromise — it is compassionate wisdom in action.**

Quick Tips for Respecting Traditions While Ensuring Health:

- **Celebrate traditions mindfully** — understand the spirit, but modify practices when needed for health.

- **Consult your healthcare provider** before undertaking fasting or major dietary changes during pregnancy.

- **Involve family elders** in open conversations to create supportive environments.

- **Balance cultural foods** by ensuring they meet your daily nutritional requirements.

- **Remember: Emotional wellness matters too** — respect for traditions can bring comfort, but health must remain the top priority.

Traditions connect us to our roots, while science lights the path to a safer future. By blending both with love and awareness, you create a nurturing world where both your dreams and your baby can thrive.

CHAPTER VII: EMOTIONAL WELLNESS IN PREGNANCY: COUNSELING, SCREENING & SUPPORT

"A mother's mental well-being

is the cradle in which the future

of her child begins to take shape."

— Anonymous

Pregnancy is not only a physical transformation — it is a profound emotional journey. As a woman's body prepares to nurture new life, her mind, too, undergoes powerful shifts. Yet, mental and emotional health often remain under-addressed in routine antenatal care. This chapter sheds light on the importance of emotional wellness in pregnancy, focusing on three critical pillars: building psychological preparedness for parenthood, screening for anxiety and depression, and strengthening the role of support systems and partners. By addressing the mind alongside the body, we move closer to truly holistic maternity care.

(A) Building Emotional Readiness for Parenthood

1. Introduction

Pregnancy is often perceived as a purely physical journey, but the emotional preparation it demands is equally profound. Becoming a parent isn't just about nurturing a growing life — it is about nurturing a new identity within oneself. Emotional readiness lays the foundation for a smoother transition into parenthood, fostering resilience, adaptability, and deeper bonds between parents and their child.

2. Why Emotional Preparedness Matters

- **Mental Health Impacts Pregnancy Outcomes**: Stress, anxiety, and unresolved emotional issues can affect fetal development and maternal health.

- **Strengthens Parent-Child Bonding**: An emotionally prepared parent is better equipped for early attachment and caregiving.

- **Improves Partner Relationships**: Preparing emotionally fosters stronger communication and shared responsibility between partners.

- **Builds Parental Confidence**: Reduces fear of the unknown, minimizes postpartum emotional crises, and enhances decision-making skills.

("Studies show that maternal emotional stress during pregnancy can influence the baby's future emotional regulation and stress response mechanisms.")

3. Signs of Someone Who Might Not be Fully Emotionally Ready

- Persistent fear or denial about pregnancy.

- Overwhelming anxiety about childbirth or parenting.

- Strained partner relationships without discussion.

- Emotional numbness or detachment from the pregnancy.

- Unrealistic expectations about parenthood ("it must be perfect").

4. Simple Practices to Foster Emotional Readiness

- **Daily Self-Check-ins**: Take 5 minutes to ask, "How am I feeling about becoming a parent today?"

- **Prenatal Counseling**: Even a single session can help clarify emotions and expectations.

- **Parenting Preparation Classes**: Focused not only on labor, but also on emotional changes.

- **Bonding Exercises**: Talking, reading, or singing to the unborn baby can enhance emotional connection.

- **Building a Village**: Engaging with family, friends, or support groups to prevent emotional isolation.

5. Closing Thought

Becoming a parent begins long before *a child is placed in your arms — it begins in your heart and mind. Emotional readiness isn't about being perfectly prepared;* ***it's about being open, aware, and willing to grow alongside your baby.***

Real Life Example: The Planner Who Panicked

Scenario: Priya, a 31-year-old marketing executive, always thrived on structure. When she became pregnant, she had a detailed plan—diet, delivery date, work handover, baby names. But one day, an unexpected spotting (minimal bleeding P/V) episode sent her into a panic spiral. Despite medical reassurance, she couldn't calm her fears.

Emotional Insight: Her anxiety wasn't about the event—it was about **loss of control**. Through counseling and journaling, Priya learned that **parenting isn't about planning perfectly; it's about being emotionally adaptable**. Her readiness grew not from control, but from acceptance.

(B) Mental Health Checkpoints in Antenatal Care

"Pregnancy is not just about growing a baby,

but about growing into a new version of oneself

— emotionally, mentally, and spiritually."

— Dr. Shefali Tsabary

1. Introduction

Pregnancy is often painted as a joyful phase, but for many women, it also brings emotional turbulence. Hormonal shifts, lifestyle changes, and anticipatory stress can trigger or worsen mental health conditions. Left unchecked, prenatal anxiety and depression can impact not only the mother but also fetal development and long-term child health. **Early screening is not a luxury — it is essential care.**

2. Why Screen for Mental Health Issues in Pregnancy?

- **High Prevalence**: Studies show that **10-25%** of pregnant women experience clinically significant anxiety or depression.

- **Often Undiagnosed**: Symptoms are masked or mistaken as "normal mood swings."

- **Risks if Unchecked**:
  o Poor nutrition or antenatal care compliance
  o Higher risk of preterm labor or low birth weight
  o Increased postpartum depression risk
  o Impaired bonding with the newborn

3. Common Screening Tools Used Globally

- **EPDS (Edinburgh Postnatal Depression Scale)**
  Widely used, validated for both antenatal and postnatal periods.

- **PHQ-9 (Patient Health Questionnaire-9)**
  Measures severity of depressive symptoms.

- **GAD-7 (Generalized Anxiety Disorder Scale)**
  Evaluates anxiety intensity.
  These tools are easy-to-administer, take less than 10 minutes, and can be repeated across visits.

4. Red Flags Not to Miss (Beyond the Scales)

- Persistent sadness or guilt

- Emotional numbness or disinterest in the baby

- Excessive irritability or anger

- Social withdrawal or fear of being alone

- Sleep disturbances unrelated to physical discomfort

- Intrusive or hopeless thoughts

When in doubt, clinician should ask twice, gently. Many women won't express distress unless they feel psychologically safe.

5. Case Study for Contextual Understanding

Case:
Neha, a 28-year-old teacher in her second trimester, visited the antenatal clinic for her regular checkup. She smiled and answered everything as "normal." But when the nurse casually

asked about sleep, Neha broke down. She'd been having panic attacks at night. On administering the EPDS, she scored 15 — moderate depression. She was referred to a counselor and began therapy. Over time, her symptoms eased, and her confidence as a mother grew.

6. Action Steps After Screening

- **Mild symptoms**: Lifestyle changes, increased family support, mindfulness, group sessions.

- **Moderate symptoms**: Referral to a mental health professional, cognitive behavioral therapy (CBT).

- **Severe symptoms**: Psychiatric evaluation, risk-benefit discussion on safe pharmacologic interventions (e.g., SSRIs with obstetric guidance)

7. Closing Insight

Screening for anxiety and depression should be as routine as checking blood pressure. A mentally healthy mother is more likely to raise a mentally healthy child — and that begins with acknowledging her inner world with the same urgency as her physical health.

(C) The Power of Together: Partner and Family Support in Pregnancy

"To care for a pregnant woman's body

but ignore her mind is to build

a home on a shaky foundation".

— **Adapted Medical Saying**

1. Introduction

Behind every emotionally strong pregnant woman is often an unseen circle of support — partners, parents, friends, and caregivers. While antenatal care often focuses on the physical well-being of the mother, **emotional resilience is often born from her environment**. Support isn't just helpful — it is **protective**, buffering her from stress, enhancing confidence, and improving outcomes for both mother and baby.

2. Why Support Systems Matter in Pregnancy

- **Reduces Stress Hormones**: Women with strong emotional support show lower cortisol levels.

- **Lowers Risk of Perinatal Depression**: Emotional isolation is a major risk factor for prenatal/postpartum mental illness.

- **Improves Maternal Health Behaviors**: Encouragement leads to better nutrition, exercise, and medication adherence.

- **Enhances Bonding with the Baby**: When the mother is emotionally secure, bonding with the baby comes more naturally.

*"**Support is not just about being present; it's about being emotionally available.**"*

3. Role of the Partner: From Supporter to Co-Nurturer

- **Attend appointments**: Increases connection with both mother and unborn child.

- **Participate in childbirth education**: Prepares emotionally and practically for parenting.

- **Validate feelings**: Pregnancy hormones can intensify emotions — empathy goes a long way.

- **Plan together**: Nursery, finances, delivery preferences — sharing these lightens emotional load.

- **Be mentally present**: Emotional intimacy is a stronger shield than material gestures alone.

4. Barriers to Support and How to Overcome Them

Barrier	Possible Solutions
Unsupportive partner or family	Introduce third-party counseling
Cultural silence around emotions	Encourage prenatal group discussions
Geographical distance from family	Online support groups, community healthcare
Mental load burnout	Delegate responsibilities, engage helpers

5. Real-Time Example

Case:
Shruti, an IT professional in her third trimester, lived away from her parents and had a partner busy in work, not getting leave. She began to feel invisible. Upon speaking with her

Obstetrician, she was referred to a local pregnancy support circle. Weekly meetings became her lifeline, providing friendships and validation she desperately needed.

6. Simple Exercises to Strengthen Support

- **Partner Reflection**: Write down 5 things you're both excited or anxious about becoming parents.

- **Daily Check-in**: Ask "What was the most challenging part of your day?" every night.

- **Appoint a 'Support Champion'**: One friend or family member dedicated to weekly check-ins.

- **Build a 'Support Plan' Before Delivery**: Who will be there postpartum? Who handles meals, visitors, errands?

7. Closing Message

Pregnancy is a transformation *— not just for the mother, but for everyone around her.* ***When partners and support systems lean*** *in emotionally, not just physically, they co-create a nurturing space where new life doesn't just grow — it* ***thrives***.

CHAPTER VIII: COMMUNICATION: EMPOWERING WOMEN WITH KNOWLEDGE

"We don't just need more antenatal care.

We need earlier, smarter,

and more human antenatal care."

(A) Patient Education Strategies: Bridging the Gap Between Clinicians and Expectant Women

Pregnancy is not just a biological journey—it's an emotional, psychological, and educational transformation. Yet, in many healthcare systems, especially in developing countries, the **clinical consultations often focus on prescriptions and checklists**, leaving little room for **patient understanding or empowerment**.

Why Patient Education Matters Early

The first trimester is a window of immense importance: organogenesis, risk screenings, and nutritional foundations all begin here. However, **many women remain unaware** of the significance of early prenatal visits, often because this knowledge is never clearly communicated. The result? Missed opportunities for prevention, early diagnosis, and timely intervention.

The Current Gap

Clinicians are often overburdened. Patients are often intimidated, shy, or uninformed. This **creates a communication gap** where crucial early warnings or recommendations fall through the cracks. For example:

- Women may not understand why **folic acid before 12 weeks** is vital.

- They may believe ultrasound is only for gender detection.

- Many still think antenatal care starts after the "bump shows."

Effective Patient Education Strategies

To bridge this gap, education must become **interactive, personalized, and culturally sensitive.** Here are some proven strategies:

- **Visual Communication Tools:** Use flipcharts, animations, and pictorial leaflets, especially in rural or low-literacy settings. For example, a simple flowchart showing "what happens in the first 12 weeks" can change behavior dramatically.

- **Mobile Health (mHealth) and WhatsApp Groups:** Short, bite-sized information delivered through mobile platforms is highly effective. A 30-second video explaining what to eat in the first trimester can have more impact than a 15-minute lecture.

- **Shared Decision-Making:** Instead of prescribing care, involve the mother in **choices**: "Would you like to start folic acid now or wait for a few tests?" When women participate, they remember better and comply more.

- **Group Counseling and Peer Support Circles:** Bringing 3–5 women together for joint education sessions builds **confidence** and fosters community learning. They ask questions they might not ask in solo consultations.

- **Family Involvement** Educating spouses or mother-in-law's—who are often decision-makers in Indian households—can greatly influence care-seeking behavior. A simple video in regional language explaining "why early ANC matters" can work wonders.

Real-Life Example

In a community-based health project in Maharashtra, the introduction of short videos shown on tablet devices during home visits increased early ANC registrations by 40% in 6 months. Why? Because the message was **accessible, visual, and repeated**.

Takeaway Message

*Bridging the gap in communication doesn't require revolutionary tools. It needs **consistent, human-centered strategies** that meet the woman where she is—emotionally, socially, and intellectually. **Empowered patients** are the strongest allies for better outcomes.*

(B) Guidelines and Recommendations: FIGO, ACOG, WHO — What They Say About Early Antenatal Care

When it comes to maternal health, **global health organizations speak in one voice**: **start antenatal care early and meaningfully**. Yet, the disconnect between **guidelines and ground reality** often persists—especially in underserved regions.

1. WHO (World Health Organization)

Key Recommendation: In its 2016 update, WHO recommends **a minimum of 8 antenatal visits**, with the **first visit ideally before 12 weeks of gestation**.

Why this matters:

- **Earlier visit = Earlier detection** of high-risk pregnancies, infections, and nutritional deficiencies.

- **More visits** = Better communication, stronger trust, **improved outcomes.**

Unique Contribution: WHO emphasizes **continuity of care** and **respectful maternity services**, placing **empathy and access** at the heart of antenatal care—not just procedures.

2. ACOG (American College of Obstetricians and Gynecologists)

Key Recommendation: Initiate prenatal care in the **first trimester**—ideally **by 10 weeks**.

Why this matters:

- Early screening for **aneuploidy, gestational diabetes, preeclampsia risk.**

- Early discussion of **lifestyle, medications, vaccinations, and mental health.**

Unique Contribution: ACOG supports **personalized risk-based care**, suggesting that not all pregnancies require the same pathway—but **all should begin with the same urgency.**

3. FIGO (International Federation of Gynecology and Obstetrics)

Key Recommendation: FIGO highlights the need for **"Preconception and Early Pregnancy Interventions"** to achieve better global maternal and child health outcomes.

Why this matters:

- FIGO emphasizes the **"first 1,00 days or the first trimester"** as a golden window of opportunity to address health risks, establish healthy habits to improve outcomes for both the mother and the developing baby. FIGO stresses the importance of preconception care.

- **FIGO's Preconception Checklist:** FIGO has developed a checklist to help healthcare providers and women prepare for pregnancy, emphasizing the importance of this period for long term health.

- Calls for **integrating nutrition, mental health, and genetics** into routine antenatal visits.

- **Early Detection of Risks:** Screening during the first 100 days can identify and address potential risks like pre-eclampsia, and gestational diabetes, which can have long term implications for both the mother and child.

Unique Contribution: FIGO promotes **multidisciplinary team approaches** and **health system strengthening** for sustained early ANC success.

How These Guidelines Align with my Book's Message:

*All three institutions recognize the **first trimester as a critical window**—for diagnosis, for education, and for intervention. My book—**Revisiting Antenatal Care**—embodies this global consensus but contextualizes it in the **real-world barriers and behavioral shifts** needed to implement these ideals.*

It's one thing to have a guideline. It's another to **make it real in a village in Bihar or an urban slum in Nairobi**. That's why this chapter doesn't stop at quoting policies—but prepares the ground for the next subchapter: **"Challenges in Implementation in Developing Countries."**

(C) Challenges in Implementation: The Roadblocks in Developing Countries

Global recommendations may be crystal clear, but when the **rubber meets the rural road**, implementation becomes a different story. In many developing countries, including India, the journey from **policy to practice** is riddled with obstacles— some visible, others deeply systemic.

This subchapter examines the **practical, cultural, economic, and infrastructural barriers** that hinder timely and effective antenatal care in low- and middle-income countries (LMICs).

1. Awareness Deficit: The First Barrier is Invisible

Many women, especially in rural and tribal areas, are unaware that antenatal care **even begins in the first trimester**. They associate healthcare visits with visible symptoms or complications—not preventive well-being.

A mother in a Jharkhand village once said, "Why visit the doctor when the baby isn't even showing?"

This mindset reflects a **generational gap in maternal health education.**

2. Access and Infrastructure

- Long distances to healthcare centers

- Lack of transportation or funds for travel

- Overburdened and under-equipped primary health centers.

In some regions, **only one nurse or ANM serves hundreds of households**, making regular, early checkups nearly impossible.

3. Workforce Challenges

Skilled healthcare providers are often concentrated in urban hospitals. Rural clinics may lack doctors, lab facilities, or even basic ultrasound equipment. Even where services exist, **overwork, poor pay, and burnout** lead to less empathetic care delivery.

4. Cultural and Social Barriers

- **Patriarchal norms** may prevent women from seeking care without male or elder approval.

- Superstitions about "hiding" pregnancy in early months still exist.

- **Mistrust** toward government facilities or modern medicine due to past experiences.

5. Economic Constraints

Even where antenatal services are nominally free, **indirect costs** (transport, lost wages, informal payments) deter early registration. A day's labor lost is a meal lost for many households.

6. Digital Divide and Health Literacy

While mobile health (mHealth) is growing, many communities lack **digital literacy** or even basic mobile access. Health information shared through apps or WhatsApp doesn't reach **the last mile.**

7. Policy Gaps and Delays

Some regions are yet to fully adopt the **8-visit WHO model**, and local policies often lag behind global recommendations.

Where policies exist, they may not be monitored or evaluated effectively.

Real-World Example

In a slum near Nairobi, a mobile clinic introduced **free first-trimester screenings**. Uptake increased briefly but plateaued because women **didn't receive follow-ups or clear communication**. **The message:** infrastructure alone isn't enough—**sustained engagement and trust-building** are key.

Moving Forward

*The next logical step? Explore what the **future of early antenatal care** could and should look like in a rapidly changing world—where **AI, telemedicine, behavioral science, and policy innovation** may finally close the gap.*

(D) The Future of Early Antenatal Care: Innovation, Integration, and Inclusion

As we stand at the crossroads of **medicine and technology**, the future of antenatal care is no longer just about when women visit—but **how, where, and with what support** they receive care. The first trimester is gaining the attention it always deserved, and tomorrow's maternal health landscape is poised to be **smarter, more personalized, and more accessible**.

This subchapter envisions the **future of early antenatal care**—driven by innovation, equity, and woman-centered design.

1. AI & Predictive Analytics: Risk Detection, Reimagined

Imagine a system that doesn't wait for complications—but **predicts them**.

AI-driven apps can analyze baseline data (BP, BMI, family history) to flag women at high risk for **preeclampsia, gestational diabetes**, or anemia—*before* symptoms arise.

Tools like **SFlt-1/PlGF ratios** or first-trimester biochemical markers will become routine, automated, and affordable.

AI chatbots may even offer **24/7 guidance**, helping bridge the doctor-patient communication gap in underserved areas.

2. Telemedicine & Virtual ANC Clinics

- Women in remote areas can consult specialists via **teleconsultation**, saving time, travel, and cost.

- **Community health workers** can use mobile devices to transmit vital signs, ultrasound images, and lab results for remote review.

- Virtual group classes can replace the one-size-fits-all "nutrition talk," offering **targeted support** from trimester one.

3. Personalized, Behaviorally Informed Care Pathways

Future antenatal care will no longer follow a rigid protocol. Instead, women will receive **customized care journeys** based on their:

- Health risks
- Socioeconomic status
- Emotional needs
- Personal preferences

Behavioral nudges—reminders, milestone messages, and rewards—can improve **appointment adherence and supplement compliance**.

4. Community-Integrated Models

- **Local champions**, midwives, and trained ASHA workers will continue to play a crucial role—but with more support, tech tools, and training.

- Integration with **schools, Anganwadi's, and self-help groups** will bring early ANC awareness to women even *before* they become pregnant.

5. Men's Involvement and Family-Centric Approaches

The future recognizes that a pregnant woman doesn't exist in isolation. Efforts will shift toward:

- **Partner education sessions**
- **Family-centered counseling**
- Breaking myths and empowering the *entire household* to support early pregnancy care

6. Policy Innovation and Public-Private Partnerships

Governments, NGOs, and private health tech startups will co-create models where:

- **Early ANC incentives** are tied to digital health wallets or UPI-linked platforms

- Mobile vans provide doorstep **first-trimester checkups**

- **Data privacy and consent** are built into every new tech tool

Vision for 2030 and Beyond

By 2030, early antenatal care should no longer be a privilege. It should be a universal standard, with every woman—rural or urban—receiving timely, compassionate, and evidence-based guidance from the moment her journey begins.

"We don't just need more antenatal care. We need earlier, smarter, and more human antenatal care."

CHAPTER IX: CONCLUSION: STRONG BEGINNINGS, SAFER JOURNEY

"Let this book be a nudge—to think earlier, act earlier, and care earlier. Because when you strengthen the beginning, you change the entire story"

Pregnancy is often described as a journey—but like every journey, its **outcome depends on where and how it begins**. For far too long, antenatal care has focused heavily on the second and third trimesters, when complications are already unfolding. But as the science, stories, and strategies in this book have shown, the **real power to transform outcomes lies in the first trimester—or even before**.

This book, ***Revisiting Antenatal Care,*** is not just a medical reflection—it's a call to rewire our thinking. It challenges the traditional pyramid of care and turns it upside down, placing **early care at the foundation, not the fringe.**

What We've Learned

- The **first trimester is not a waiting period**—it's a window of action.
- Modern tools—**from genetic screening to AI-based risk detection**—can only be effective if deployed early.
- Empowering women with **clear, culturally sensitive communication** can bridge the fatal gap between knowledge and care.
- Global guidelines from WHO, ACOG, and FIGO already emphasize early action—but **implementation in developing nations needs innovation, empathy, and equity.**
- The future of antenatal care will be **data-driven, personalized, community-based, and inclusive.**

Why This Matters Now More Than Ever

In an age where maternal deaths are preventable, and congenital anomalies are detectable, **delaying care is no longer an option—it's a disservice.** Every missed folic acid tablet, every skipped first-trimester visit, and every unspoken concern can ripple into lifelong consequences—for the mother, the baby, and society at large.

A Collective Responsibility

This is not a gynecologist's job alone.
This is not a woman's burden alone.
This is **everyone's mission**—from community workers to policymakers, educators to family members. The moment a pregnancy is confirmed—or even suspected—should trigger **a cascade of support, guidance, and medical care**.

A Vision for the Future

Let us imagine a world where:

- Every woman knows **why the first 12 weeks matter most.**
- No woman hesitates to seek care because of distance, stigma, or ignorance.
- Every clinician sees not just a patient—but a mother with a future in her womb.

That is the future we must work and look forward for the revolution that begins in the first trimester.

In summary, you don't need big changes to make a big difference. Sometimes, the most profound impact comes from revisiting what we thought we knew, and re-aligning it with what truly matters. Let this book be a nudge—to think earlier, act earlier, and care earlier. Because when you strengthen the beginning, you change the entire story.

CHAPTER X: REFERENCES

1.A comprehensive assessment of preconception health needs and interventions regarding women of childbearing age: a systematic review. Zaçe D, Orfino A, Mariaviteritti A, Versace V, Ricciardi W, DI Pietro ML. J Prev Med Hyg. 2022; 63:0–99. doi: 10.15167/2421-4248/jpmh2022.63.1.2391. [DOI] [PMC free article] [PubMed] [Google Scholar]

2.Preconception care for improving perinatal outcomes: the time to act. Atrash HK, Johnson K, Adams M, Cordero JF, Howse J. Matern Child Health J. 2006;10:0–11. doi: 10.1007/s10995-006-0100-4. [DOI] [PMC free article] [PubMed] [Google Scholar]

3.Institute of Medicine (US) Committee on Improving Birth Outcomes. In: Reducing birth defects: meeting the challenge in the developing world. Washington, D.C: National Academies Press (US); 2003. Impact and patterns of occurrence; pp. 22–67. [PubMed] [Google Scholar]

4.2.5 million annual deaths-are neonates in low- and middle-income countries too small to be seen? A bottom-up overview on neonatal morbi-mortality. Rosa-Mangeret F, Benski AC, Golaz A, et al. Trop Med Infect Dis. 2022;7:64. doi: 10.3390/tropicalmed7050064. [DOI] [PMC free article] [PubMed] [Google Scholar]

5.Preconception care: closing the gap in the continuum of care to accelerate improvements in maternal, newborn and child health. Dean SV, Lassi ZS, Imam AM, Bhutta ZA. Reprod Health. 2014;11 Suppl 3:0. doi: 10.1186/1742-4755-11-S3-S1. [DOI] [PMC free article] [PubMed] [Google Scholar]

6.Preconception care: delivery strategies and packages for care. Lassi ZS, Dean SV, Mallick D, Bhutta ZA. Reprod

Health. 2014;11 Suppl 3:0. doi: 10.1186/1742-4755-11-S3-S7. [DOI] [PMC free article] [PubMed] [Google Scholar]

7.Before the beginning: nutrition and lifestyle in the preconception period and its importance for future health. Stephenson J, Heslehurst N, Hall J, et al. Lancet. 2018;391:1830–1841. doi: 10.1016/S0140-6736(18)30311-8. [DOI] [PMC free article] [PubMed] [Google Scholar]

8.In: Mother to baby | fact sheets [internet] Brentwood, TN: Organization of Teratology Information Specialists (OTIS); 2021. Critical periods of development. [PubMed] [Google Scholar]

9.Preconception care (position paper) [Jun; 2023]. 2023. https://www.aafp.org/about/policies/all/preconceptioncare.html https://www.aafp.org/about/policies/all/preconception-care.html

10.Family planning/contraception methods. [Jun; 2023]. 2023. 2023] https://www.who.int/news-room/fact-sheets/detail/family-planning-contraception

11.Managing preexisting diabetes for pregnancy: summary of evidence and consensus recommendations for care. Kitzmiller JL, Block JM, Brown FM, et al. Diabetes Care. 2008;31:1060–1079. doi: 10.2337/dc08-9020. [DOI] [PMC free article] [PubMed] [Google Scholar]

12.Genetic counseling. [Jun; 2023]. 2023. https://www.cdc.gov/genomics/gtesting/genetic_counseling.htm https://www.cdc.gov/genomics/gtesting/genetic_counseling.htm

13.Vaccines and immunization: what is vaccination? [Jun; 2023]. 2023. https://www.who.int/news-room/questions-and-answers/item/vaccines-and-immunization-what-is-vaccination https://www.who.int/news-room/questions-and-answers/item/vaccines-and-immunization-what-is-vaccination

14.Mental health promotion and illness prevention: a challenge for psychiatrists. Min JA, Lee CU, Lee C. Psychiatry Investig. 2013;10:307–316. doi: 10.4306/pi.2013.10.4.307. [DOI] [PMC free article] [PubMed] [Google Scholar]

15.Implementation of preconception care for women with diabetes. Yehuda I. Diabetes Spectr. 2016;29:105–114. doi: 10.2337/diaspect.29.2.105. [DOI] [PMC free article] [PubMed] [Google Scholar]

16.Paternal preconception modifiable risk factors for adverse pregnancy and offspring outcomes: a review of contemporary evidence from observational studies. Carter T, Schoenaker D, Adams J, Steel A. BMC Public Health. 2023;23:509. doi: 10.1186/s12889-023-15335-1. [DOI] [PMC free article] [PubMed] [Google Scholar]

17.Prevention and early intervention in youth mental health: is it time for a multidisciplinary and trans-diagnostic model for care? Colizzi M, Lasalvia A, Ruggeri M. Int J Ment Health Syst. 2020;14:23. doi: 10.1186/s13033-020-00356-9. [DOI] [PMC free article] [PubMed] [Google Scholar]

18.Born too soon: care before and between pregnancy to prevent preterm births: from evidence to action. Dean SV, Mason E, Howson CP, Lassi ZS, Imam AM, Bhutta ZA. Reprod Health. 2013;10 Suppl 1:0. doi: 10.1186/1742-4755-10-S1-S3. [DOI] [PMC free article] [PubMed] [Google Scholar]

19.The importance of nutrition in pregnancy and lactation: lifelong consequences. Marshall NE, Abrams B, Barbour LA, et al. Am J Obstet Gynecol. 2022;226:607–632. doi: 10.1016/j.ajog.2021.12.035. [DOI] [PMC free article] [PubMed] [Google Scholar]

20.Cognitive behavioral therapy for substance use disorders. McHugh RK, Hearon BA, Otto MW. Psychiatr Clin North Am. 2010;33:511–525. doi: 10.1016/j.psc.2010.04.012. [DOI] [PMC free article] [PubMed] [Google Scholar]

21.Planning for Pregnancy | Preconception Care | CDC. Centers for Disease Control and Prevention. [Jun; 2023]. 2023. https://www.cdc.gov/preconception/planning.html https://www.cdc.gov/preconception/planning.html

22.Preconception care and genetic risk: ethical issues. De Wert GM, Dondorp WJ, Knoppers BM. J Community Genet. 2012;3:221–228. doi: 10.1007/s12687-011-0074-9. [DOI] [PMC free article] [PubMed] [Google Scholar]

23.Guidelines for vaccinating pregnant women. [Jun; 2023]. 2023. https://www.cdc.gov/vaccines/pregnancy/hcp-toolkit/guidelines.html https://www.cdc.gov/vaccines/pregnancy/hcp-toolkit/guidelines.html

24.Preconception mental health predicts pregnancy complications and adverse birth outcomes: a national population-based study. Witt WP, Wisk LE, Cheng ER, Hampton JM, Hagen EW. Matern Child Health J. 2012;16:1525–1541. doi: 10.1007/s10995-011-0916-4. [DOI] [PMC free article] [PubMed] [Google Scholar]

25.Neural tube defects, folic acid and methylation. Imbard A, Benoist JF, Blom HJ. Int J Environ Res Public Health. 2013;10:4352–4389. doi: 10.3390/ijerph10094352. [DOI] [PMC free article] [PubMed] [Google Scholar]

26.Cardiac changes in infants of diabetic mothers. Al-Biltagi M, El Razaky O, El Amrousy D. World J Diabetes. 2021;12:1233–1247. doi: 10.4239/wjd.v12.i8.1233. [DOI] [PMC free article] [PubMed] [Google Scholar]

27.CDC grand rounds: public health strategies to prevent preterm birth. Shapiro-Mendoza CK, Barfield WD, Henderson Z, James A, Howse JL, Iskander J, Thorpe PG. MMWR Morb Mortal Wkly Rep. 2016;65:826–830. doi: 10.15585/mmwr.mm6532a4. [DOI] [PubMed] [Google Scholar]

28.Optimizing nutrition in preterm low birth weight infants-consensus summary. Kumar RK, Singhal A, Vaidya U, Banerjee S, Anwar F, Rao S. Front Nutr. 2017;4:20. doi: 10.3389/fnut.2017.00020. [DOI] [PMC free article] [PubMed] [Google Scholar]

29.Genetic screening: a primer for primary care. Andermann A,Blancquaert. https://www.ncbi.nlm.nih.gov/pmc/articles/ PMC2860823/ Can Fam Physician. 2010;56:333–339. [PMC free article] [PubMed] [Google Scholar]

30.Preconception care: advancing from 'important to do and can be done' to 'is being done and is making a difference'. Mason E, Chandra-Mouli V, Baltag V, Christiansen C, Lassi ZS, Bhutta ZA. Reprod Health. 2014;11 Suppl 3:0. doi: 10.1186/1742-4755-11-S3-S8. [DOI] [PMC free article] [PubMed] [Google Scholar]

31.Preconceptional care: a systematic review of the current situation and recommendations for the future. Braspenningx S, Haagdorens M, Blaumeiser B, Jacquemyn Y, Mortier G. https://www.ncbi.nlm.nih.gov/pmc/articles/PMC398735 1/ Facts Views Vis Obgyn. 2013;5:13–25. [PMC free article] [PubMed] [Google Scholar]

32. *"How Are Thalassemias Diagnosed?"*. NHLBI. 3 July 2012. *Archived* from the original on 16 September 2016. Retrieved 5 September 2016.

33.Jump up to:[a] [b] *"How Are Thalassemias Treated?"*. NHLBI. 3 July 2012. *Archived* from the original on 16 September 2016. Retrieved 5 September 2016.

34._Vos T, Allen C, Arora M, Barber RM, Bhutta ZA, Brown A, et al. (GBD 2015 Disease and Injury Incidence and Prevalence Collaborators) (October 2016). "Global, regional, and national incidence, prevalence, and years lived with disability for 310 diseases and injuries, 1990-2015: a systematic analysis for the Global Burden of Disease Study 2015"._ Lancet. **388** (10053): 1545–1602. _doi:10.1016/S0140-6736(16)31678-6. PMC 5055577. PMID 27733282._

35._Wang H, Naghavi M, Allen C, Barber RM, Bhutta ZA, Carter A, et al. (GBD 2015 Mortality and Causes of Death Collaborators) (October 2016). "Global, regional, and national life expectancy, all-cause mortality, and cause-specific mortality for 249 causes of death, 1980-2015: a systematic analysis for the Global Burden of Disease Study 2015"._ Lancet. **388** (10053): 1459–1544. _doi:10.1016/s0140-6736(16)31012-1. PMC 5388903. PMID 27733281._

36.Jump up to:_[a] [b] [c] "What is Thalassemia?"._ National Heart, Lung, and Blood Institute (NHLBI). 31 May 2022. Retrieved 9 December 2024.

37._"How Can Thalassemias Be Prevented?"._ NHLBI. 3 July 2012. _Archived from the original on 16 September 2016._ Retrieved 5 September 2016.

38.Corsello G, Giuffre M. Congenital malformations. J Matern Fetal Neonatal Med. 2012;1:25-29. [DOI] [PubMed] [Google Scholar]

39. Patel ZM, Adhia RA. Birth defects surveillance study. Indian J Pediatr. 2005;72:489-491. [DOI] [PubMed] [Google Scholar]

40.Obu HA, Chinawa JM, Uleanya ND, Adimora GN, Obi IE. Congenital malformations among newborns admitted in the neonatal unit of a tertiary hospital in Enugu, South-East

Nigeri: a retrospective study. BMC Res Notes. 2012;5:177. 10.1186/1756-0500-5-177 [DOI] [PMC free article] [PubMed] [Google Scholar]

41. Ajao AE, Adeoye IA. Prevalence, risk factors and outcome of congenital anomalies among neonatal admissions in Ogbomoso, Nigeria. BMC Pediatr. 2019;19(1):88. 10.1186/s12887-019-1471-1 [DOI] [PMC free article] [PubMed] [Google Scholar]

42. Fajolu IB, Ezenwa B, Akintan P, Ezeaka A. 8 years review of major congenital abnormalities in a tertiary hospital in lagos, Nigeria. Niger J Paediatr. 2016;43:175-1. [Google Scholar]

43. Lemmens M, van Vugt JMG, Willemsen M, van der Voorn P, van Bokhoven H, ten Donkelaar HJ. Causes of congenital malformations. In: Ten Donkelaar HJ, Lammens M, Hori A, eds. Clinical Neuroembryology. 2nd ed. Springer; 2014:105-164. [Google Scholar]

44. Spencer K. Aneuploidy screening in the first trimester. Am J Med Genet C Semin Med Genet. 2007;145:18–32. doi: 10.1002/ajmg.c.30119. [DOI] [PubMed] [Google Scholar]

45. Sonek J. First trimester ultrasonography in screening and detection of fetal anomalies. Am J Med Genet C Semin Med Genet. 2007;145:45–61. doi: 10.1002/ajmg.c.30120. [DOI] [PubMed] [Google Scholar]

46. Cicero S, Avgidou K, Rembouskos G, Kagan KO, et al. Nasal bone in first-trimester screening for trisomy 21. Am J Obstet Gynecol. 2006;195:109–114. doi: 10.1016/j.ajog.2005.12.057. [DOI] [PubMed] [Google Scholar]

47. Makrydimas G, Sotiriadis A, Huggon IC, Simpson J, et al. Nuchal translucency and fetal cardiac defects: a pooled analysis of major fetal echocardiography centers. Am J

Obstet Gynecol. 2005;192(1):89–95. doi: 10.1016/j.ajog.2004.06.081. [DOI] [PubMed] [Google Scholar]

48.Wapner R, Thom E, Simpson JL, Pergament E, et al. First-trimester screening for trisomies 21 and 18. N Engl J Med. 2003;349:1405–1413. doi: 10.1056/NEJMoa025273. [DOI] [PubMed] [Google Scholar]

49.Sharma G, McCullough LB, Chervenak FA. Ethical considerations of early (first vs. second trimester) risk assessment disclosure for trisomy 21 and patient choice in screening versus diagnostic testing. Am J Med Genet C Semin Med Genet. 2007;145:99–104. doi: 10.1002/ajmg.c.30118. [DOI] [PubMed] [Google Scholar]

50.Platt LD, Greene N, Johnson A, Zachary J, et al. Sequential pathways of testing after first-trimester screening for trisomy 21. Obstet Gynecol. 2004;104:661–666. doi: 10.1097/01.AOG.0000139832.79658.b9. [DOI] [PubMed] [Google Scholar]

Previous Books Published in the Series, "Women's Health"

All books are available on Amazon.in as well as on Amazon.com.

Universal Link for amazon.com:

https://relinks.me/B0BW6ZVMXY

1. **Preconception Care Makes a Difference**

"Preconception Care and Counselling is the window of opportunity to tackle all unhealthy maternal problems resulting in favorable environment for the growth of embryo/fetus."

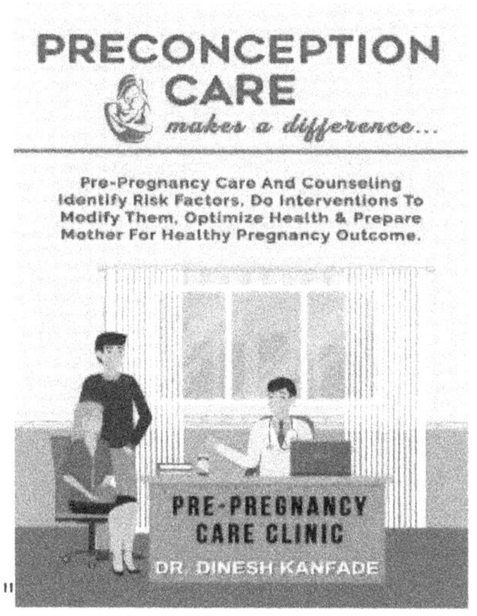

2. Understanding Menopause

"The biggest achievement of the last century is greater longevity that has resulted in an increased aged population worldwide. But the advantage of increased longevity is only when it is translated into healthy aging. Discover the secrets for understanding and managing menopause, thereby improving quality of life with this comprehensive updated guide."

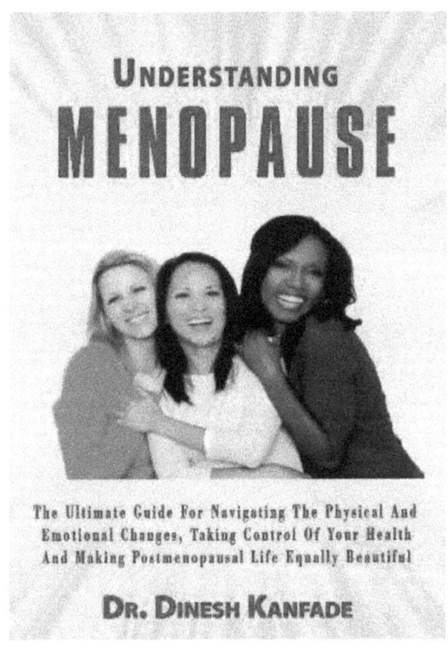

3. Heart and Bone Health

"We are living in aged population worldwide. It is obvious that women live significant part of their life after menopause. The ovaries of long years of dedicated service, have not the ability of retiring gracefully. But because of estrogen deficiency, ovaries become irritable and transmits this irritation to various organs of the body resulting in non-communicable diseases such as cardiovascular disease and osteoporosis. The advantage of increased longevity is only when it is translated into healthy aging. With a healthy lifestyle and understanding the pathophysiology of cardiovascular disease and osteoporosis in postmenopausal women, not only years will be added to increase the lifespan, but the extra years added will be of good quality. Discover the secretes of managing heart and bone health in postmenopausal women, thereby improving quality of life with this comprehensive guide."

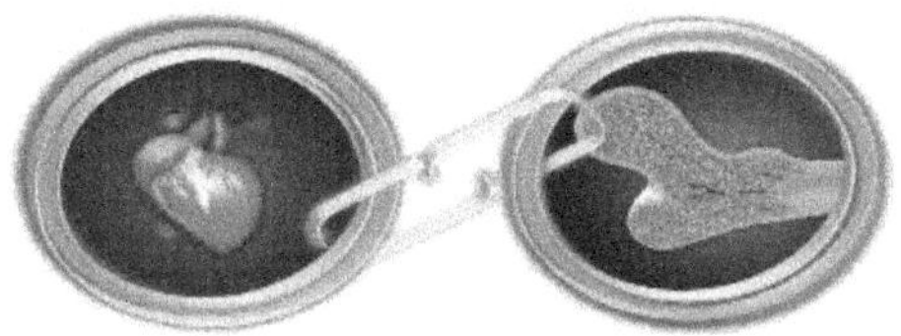

4. Embracing Postmenopausal Intimacy

"The postmenopausal phase, with its unique challenges and opportunities stands as a testament to the resilience of human intimacy. It is within this period of transformation that find an invitation to redefine and to rediscover physical closeness. Don't miss out on the transformative wisdom within these pages. Embrace the journey towards vibrant and fulfilling postmenopausal intimacy."

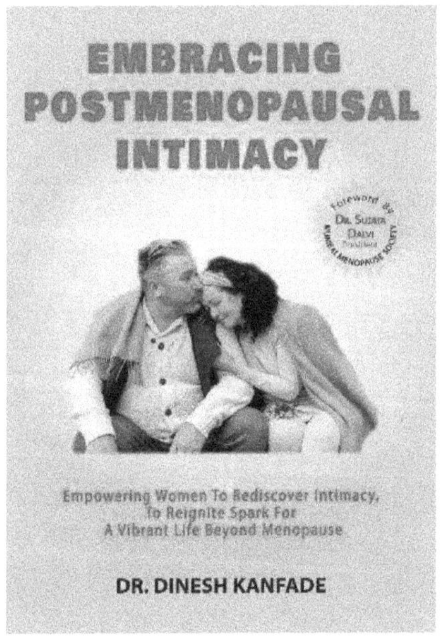

5. Menstrual Health and Hygiene

Unlock the secrets to optimal menstrual health and hygiene in this comprehensive guide.
From debunking myths to empowering insights, this book offers practical tips and evidence-based strategies for every stage of menstruation.

Whether you are seeking solutions for menstrual discomfort, navigating hygiene products or simply aiming for a healthier menstrual cycle, this book has covered everything you want in relation to menstruation.

Together, let us embark on this journey of enlightment, guided by the wisdom contained within these pages.

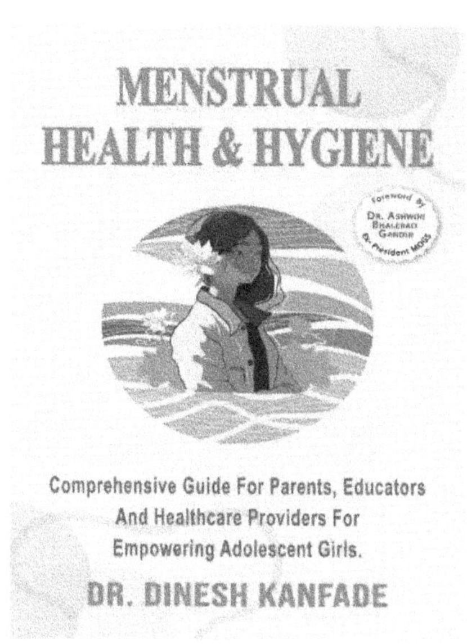

6. The Silent Struggles: Understanding Women's Mental Health

Mental health is often a quiet battle, and for women, it is a journey through the unique challenges at every stage of life.

The book is a comprehensive exploration of the emotional and psychological hurdles women face- from adolescence, through their reproductive years, to menopause.

The recurrence of heinous acts such as recent physical and sexual assault of junior doctor R. G. Kar Medical College Kolkata (August 2024), the infamous Nirbhaya case (2012) and many others suggest several concerning ground realities.

This book offers a profound understanding of how social, cultural and biological factors shape a woman's mental health.

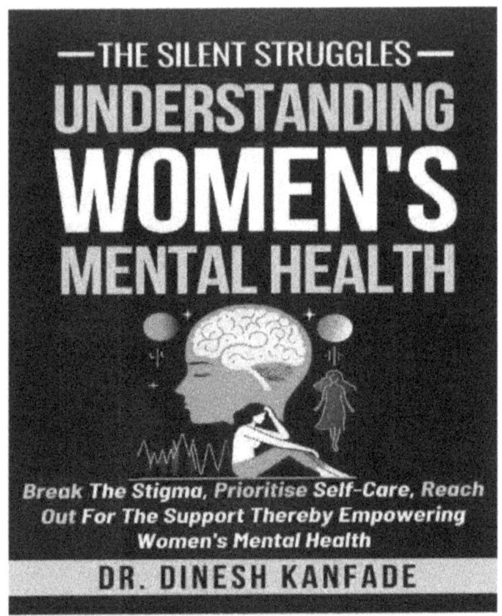

7. Nurturing Wellness: The Path to Breast Cancer Awareness

The breast has always been the symbol of womanhood and ultimate fertility. As a result, both disease and surgery of the breast evoke a fear of mutilation and loss of femininity.

Breast cancer remains a major health concern due to its high incidence worldwide and the significant impact it has on women's health.

This book contains vital information about the prevalence, prevention and tips for early detection of breast cancer for better survival rates.

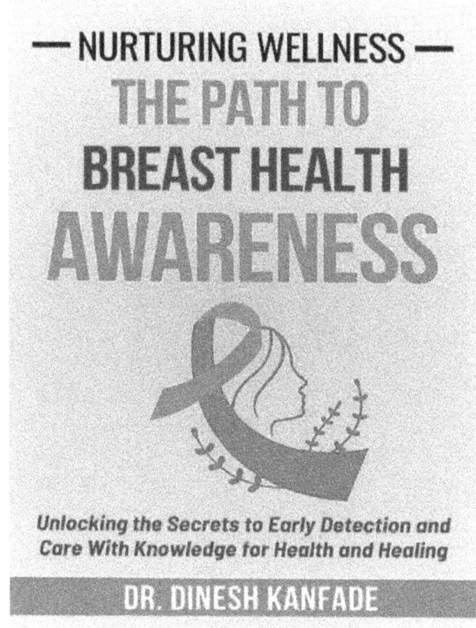

8. Nurturing Wellness: The Path to Postmenopausal Heart Disease Awareness

The biggest achievement of the last century is greater longevity that has resulted in increasing aged population worldwide. It is obvious that women have to live significant part of their lives after menopause. Menopause transition brings profound hormonal changes that can affect multiple aspects of health, including an often-overlooked issue: cardiovascular disease (CVD). Heart disease is the leading cause of death among women in postmenopausal age group, cancer being second. Yet many women are unaware of the heightened risk of CVD they face after menopause. The benefit of increased lifespan is only when it is translated into healthy aging.

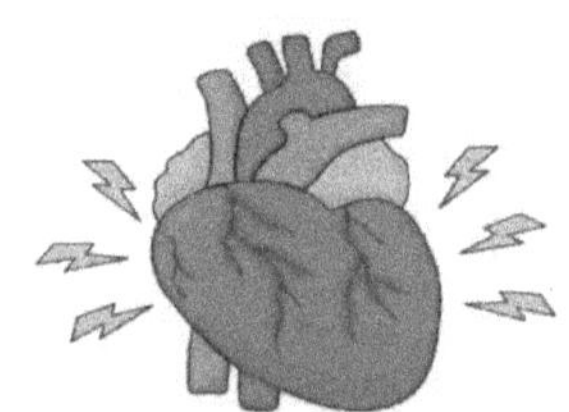

7. Nurturing Wellness: The Path to Postmenopausal Osteoporosis Awareness

Osteoporosis is frequently called the "Silent Killer" because it itself has no symptoms. The patients are unaware of their bone loss until they experience a fracture.

With aging, bone density naturally decreases in both genders, but for many women, this process accelerates after menopause due to estrogen deficiency, leading to brittle bones, subsequent fractures, and a significant impact on quality of life. Despite its widespread prevalence, osteoporosis remains an often-overlooked health issue, overshadowed by other conditions.

The rapid bone loss typically starts within the first 5 - 7 years after menopause, with women losing up to 20% of their bone mass during this period.

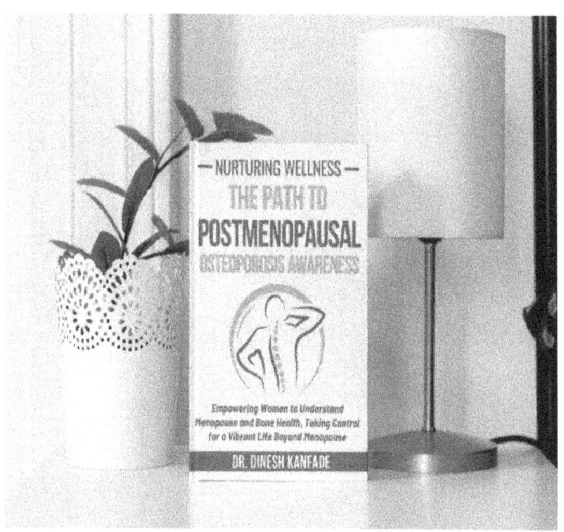

10. Demystifying Menopausal Hormone Therapy

Menopause is a natural phase in every woman's life, yet it often comes with confusion, fear, and unanswered questions—especially regarding hormone therapy. **"Demystified Menopause Hormone Therapy"** is a transformative guide that breaks down the myths and misconceptions surrounding Menopause Hormone Therapy (MHT), offering clear, evidence-based insights for women and medical practitioners alike.

Authored by a seasoned gynecologist, this book delves into the latest research on MHT, addressing its safety, benefits, and practical application. It provides tailored guidance for women with diabetes, hypertension, and other conditions, empowering them to make informed decisions.

Whether you're navigating menopause, supporting a loved one, or offering professional care, this book is your trusted companion in understanding and embracing the journey of menopause with confidence and clarity

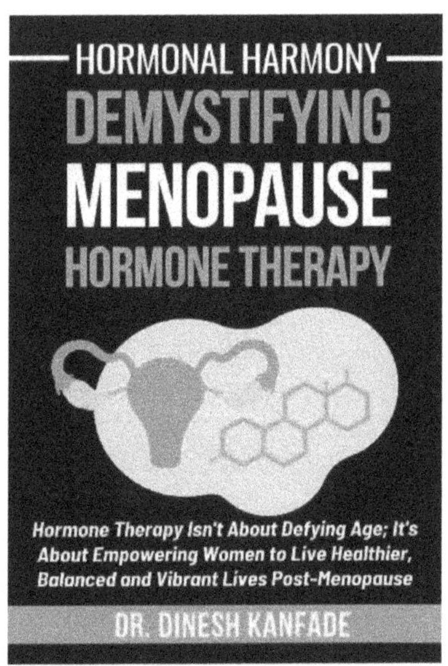

11. Women's Health Through the Lens of Ikigai

With practical tips, scientific insights, and real-life applications of Ikigai, **this book helps women cultivate longevity, vitality, and inner peace.** It provides tools to build daily habits that align with personal well-being, reduce stress, and create a fulfilling life beyond just physical health.

Whether you're a young woman looking to establish a strong foundation, a mother balancing responsibility, or someone navigating the transitions of menopause, *"Women's Health Through the Lens of Ikigai"* is your roadmap to a healthier, happier, and more meaningful life.

A must-read for women, healthcare professionals, and wellness seekers who believe in the power of purpose-driven health and holistic well-being.

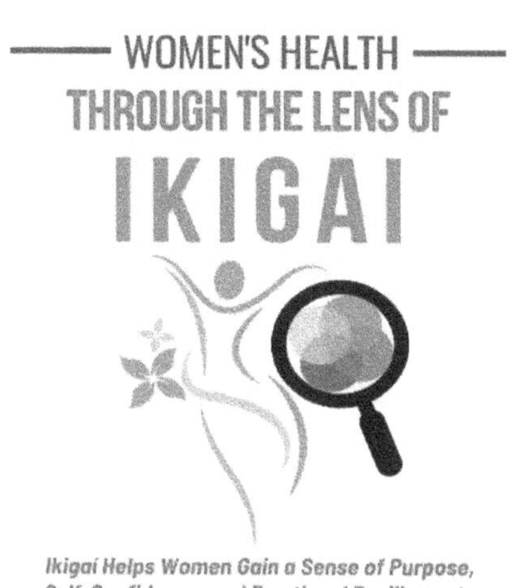

www.ingramcontent.com/pod-product-compliance
Lightning Source LLC
Chambersburg PA
CBHW040757120726

48005CB00012B/1208